CREATIVE
LONG–TERM CARE
ADMINISTRATION

CREATIVE LONG-TERM CARE ADMINISTRATION

Second Edition

Edited by

GEORGE KENNETH GORDON, ED.D.

and

RUTH STRYKER, M.A.

Associate Professors
Center for Long-Term Care Administration
Division of Health Services Administration
School of Public Health
University of Minnesota
Minneapolis, Minnesota

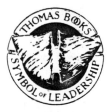

CHARLES C THOMAS • PUBLISHER
Springfield • Illinois • U.S.A.

Published and Distributed Throughout the World by

CHARLES C THOMAS • PUBLISHER
2600 South First Street
Springfield, Illinois 62717

© *1988 by* CHARLES C THOMAS • PUBLISHER

ISBN 0-398-05436-3

Library of Congress Catalog Card Number: 87-18177
First Edition, 1983

With THOMAS BOOKS *careful attention is given to all details of manufacturing
and design. It is the Publisher's desire to present books that are satisfactory as to their
physical qualities and artistic possibilities and appropriate for their particular use.*
THOMAS BOOKS *will be true to those laws of quality that assure a good name
and good will.*

Printed in the United States of America
SC-R-3

Library of Congress Cataloging-in-Publication Data

Creative long-term care administration.

    Includes bibliographies and indexes.
    1. Long-term care facilities—Administration.
I. Gordon, George Kenneth. II. Stryker, Ruth Perin.
[DNLM: 1. Long Term Care—organization & administration.
2. Nursing Homes—organization & administration.
3. Skilled Nursing Facilities—organization & administra-
tion.   Wt 30 C912]
RA999.A35C74   1988   362.1'6   87-18177
ISBN 0-398-05436-3

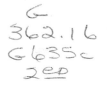

CONTRIBUTORS

JOAN ABRAHAMSON, MSW, ACSW, social worker, Sister Kenny Institute and social work consultant in long-term care, Minneapolis, Minnesota.

BARBARA PORTNOY BARRON, LNHA, MHA, Regional Vice President, Pleasant Valley Health Services, Inc., Decatur, Georgia.

MARGARET CHRISTENSON, OTR, MPH, Geriatric Environmental Concepts, Minneapolis, Minnesota.

JUDY EGGLESTON, LNHA, OTR, MPH, Director, Occupational Therapy, University of Minnesota Hospitals, Minneapolis, Minnesota.

GEORGE KENNETH GORDON, EdD, Associate Professor and Coordinator, Center for Long Term Care Administration, School of Public Health, Minneapolis, Minnesota.

RUTH HASTINGS, OTR, BS, formerly Activities Specialist, Beverly Enterprises, Northern Division, Minneapolis, Minnesota.

WILLIAM F. HENRY, MA, Administrator, International Diabetes Center, Minneapolis, Minnesota.

GEARY W. OLSEN, DVM, MPH, Epidemiologist, DOW Chemical, Health and Environmental Sciences, Midland, Michigan.

JOSEPH S. QUIGLEY, DVM, Associate Director, Center to Study Human-Animal Relationships and Environments, University of Minnesota, Minneapolis, Minnesota.

RUTH STRYKER, RN, MA, Associate Professor and Assistant Coordinator, Center for Long-Term Care Administration, School of Public Health, University of Minnesota, Minneapolis, Minnesota.

JOHN R. THOMPSON, LNHA, CAS, Executive Director, Bethany Homes, Fargo, North Dakota.

PETER THOREEN, LNHA, MHA, MA, Vice President of Operations for Riverside Medical Center, Minneapolis, Minnesota.

CAROL WOEHRER, MA, formerly instructor in long-term care administration, University of Minnesota.

PREFACE TO THE SECOND EDITION

The first edition of this book, published in 1983, has been used extensively by both graduate students and practitioners. During this five-year period, most nursing home clients have had greater disability at the time of admission and about one-third were short stay clients with intensive rehabilitation needs. The nursing home clientele of today continues to require an ever increasing level of management skill and a greater depth of professional knowledge. For this edition, the editors have made extensive changes including deletions, significant updating and major additions in an effort to assist the administrator of tomorrow.

Part I, Attitudes Affecting Organizational Outcomes in Long Term Care, contains three chapters that explore how resident outcomes are influenced by historical distortions, motivations and perceptions of often under-educated workers and disagreement of major parties on appropriate client goals.

Part II, Executive Leadership for Organizational Development, contains five chapters that explore governance, the role of the administrator, developing a management team, fiscal leadership, and special considerations of managing institutional living.

Part III, Monitoring Human Resource Management, is a new section containing major portions of *How to Reduce Employee Turnover in Nursing Homes* by Ruth Stryker (Charles C Thomas, Publisher, 1981). The chapters deals with personnel turnover as an indicator of HRM effectiveness, personnel recruitment, screening and selection, staff development, personnel policies and monitoring and evaluating HR practices.

Part IV, Creating the Environment for Health Care, discusses five contributors to the health of clients; medicine, nursing, social work, activities, and the environment.

Part V, Creating the Environment for Living, explores children and pets in the environment, support and participation of families, and dealing with death as a part of living.

Part VI, Creating the Future, attempts to provide the administrator with knowledge and tools to guide an organization through change, the only sure future event.

RUTH STRYKER
GEORGE KENNETH GORDON

PREFACE TO THE FIRST EDITION

Perhaps the essence of sound management in any setting lies in constantly evaluating and adapting both well-established practice and newly developing ideas and technologies to the conduct of managerial work. An administrator cannot risk retaining established practices which have outlived their usefulness, nor can he or she become a dilettante dabbling in new "trendy" ideas and practices which are untested, illconceived or possibly debilitating to the vitality and effectiveness of the organization.

For these reasons, textbook authors must attempt to describe specific adaptation of established management practice and make sure that new practices have been tested and found successful. In this instance, the editors and authors, along with many colleagues, have tested the ideas presented and found them to be fundamental to the growth, scope, and image of long-term care organizations.

Long-term care administrators are faced with very special problems which require knowledge from an unusually broad array of disciplines. First, they must be good managers in the traditional sense. However, because they manage a community where mentally and physically frail persons come to live, they must also understand how the environment impacts on those who live there. An organization may purport to promote health, but actually promote dependency and withdrawal by encouraging acceptance and compliance. Therefore, the administrator must also have special knowledge of therapeutic environmental interventions. In essence, the environment is part of the treatment program and can enhance or detract from resident outcomes.

During the past six years, the editors have had the privilege of working with over ninety nursing home administrators from sixteen states who were engaged in graduate study at the University of Minnesota while they continued their employment as administrators. We developed the curriculum along with initial inquiry into our many questions about the field. Subsequently, administrator/students developed more questions and embarked on major projects in their own organizations to seek some answers.

This book is based on the partnership that developed with these practicing administrators, some of whom are authors of chapters. We have learned together that the administrator, by modelling attitudes and developing creative programming, is the key to creating an outstanding nursing home. If nursing homes are to take their rightful place as specialized health care organizations in the 80s and 90s, success will require the administrator to carve out a role that takes into account an understanding and analysis of the environment—residents, families, personnel drawn to work with this clientele, financial constraints, and general attitudes that reflect fear of aging, debilitation, and death.

This book is written for teachers, students, administrators, board members, owners and health care professionals who are seeking new directions in the field. The ideas are intended to provide a better understanding of the long-term care environment and to suggest ways of applying interdisciplinary knowledge for the administrator in this setting, whether the organization is free-standing or hospital-attached.

GEORGE KENNETH GORDON
RUTH STRYKER

CONTENTS

PART I
ATTITUDES AFFECTING ORGANIZATIONAL OUTCOMES IN LONG-TERM CARE

PART II
EXECUTIVE LEADERSHIP FOR ORGANIZATIONAL DEVELOPMENT

CREATIVE
LONG-TERM CARE
ADMINISTRATION

PART I

ATTITUDES AFFECTING ORGANIZATIONAL OUTCOMES IN LONG-TERM CARE

Long-term care administrators must deal with a subtle antipathy toward their organizations from a variety of sources. It is not difficult to identify some causes of these feelings and attitudes, but others are more illusive. Administrators who are aware of the many historical and societal biases of staff and families are better prepared to reduce their effects on elderly clientele.

Part I of this book attempts to analyze some of these issues so that the administrator can deal with specific rather than general interventions. Chapter 1, Historical Obstacles to Management of Nursing Homes, deals with the "roots" of nursing homes, nursing home administration, and the field of gerontology. Chapter 2, Characteristics of the Residential Care Model, examines the integration of health care in an environment that must also be a place for living and maintain psychological health. Chapter 3, Worker Motivations, Attitudes and Perceptions, examines the attitudes and perceptions regarding the aged and nursing homes by the general public with special attention to staff, families and professional service providers.

This section provides a basis of understanding of the practices found in the field and suggests some of the pitfalls and challenges that the administrator will encounter.

Chapter 1

HISTORICAL OBSTACLES TO MANAGEMENT OF NURSING HOMES

RUTH STRYKER

INTRODUCTION

E very society must find a way of dealing with its nonproductive members. Because they depend upon, rather than support other members, they are often referred to as "the poor." Historically, the poor has included the chemically dependent (inebriates), the developmentally disabled (imbeciles), the mentally ill (lunatics), the disabled (cripples), criminals and the aged. The labels attached to these groups in the past (as indicated in parentheses) contrast with those used today and reflect gradual social change which has mainly taken place during this century.

Cultural attitudes, expediency and both the capability and willingness of a society dictate how it will deal with nonproductive members. Nomadic tribes often left them behind to die, and Eskimos commonly put them on an ice flow. During the Greco-Roman era, medical attention was given only to those who could be cured, thus abandoning the disabled and aged to prevent a drain on resources. European societies tended to group "all of the poor" by isolating them in some kind of spartan housing arrangement. Primary financial responsibility, while always mixed, has shifted across the centuries from the family to the church and philanthropy, and more recently, to the public through taxes with attempts to increase family responsibility.

Cultural attitudes toward helping nonproductive members of society have also varied. The Roman privileged class cared for "unfortunates" in order to achieve a sense of individual virtue. In contrast, Maimonides, the twelfth century Jewish physician and philosopher, declared that a recipient of benefactions should be spared a sense of shame and that assistance should enable the person to help himself—a modern day rehabilitation philosophy! This contrast in motivation of the "helper" is

4

startling—one for the benefit of the benefactor, the other for the benefit of the recipient. One might note that human nature does not seem to change; both the self-righteous and the altruist are among us today.

In addition, there is often conflict between individual and collective willingness to help the poor. While some families are willing and able to care for one another, others cannot or will not. Because some children feel it is their right to inherit family money, they accept annual parental gifts without any expectation of using them to postpone welfare eligibility for their parents. Others feel no right to spend money they themselves did not earn and will use it for their parents. Some taxpayers are more concerned about welfare cheats while others are concerned about the needy. All of these people are our nursing home residents, their families, our employees and the tax payers of this country. In long-term care, we deal with value systems and motivations that differ from our own on a daily basis. You might say, "so does everyone else." True, but compared to business and other health care settings, it has a far greater impact on the financial structure, the community image, staff morale and self esteem of residents. These almost schizophrenic aspects of modern society may pose the greatest challenge to the development of more progressive methods of caring for the aged.

HISTORY OF NURSING HOMES

Saint Helena (250–330 AD) established what is probably one of the first homes for the aged (gerokomion). She was a wealthy, intelligent, Christian convert and mother of Constantine the Great. Like other early Christian "nurses" who devoted their lives to the sick and needy, she gave direct care herself. For many centuries, individual benefactors, benevolence societies and religious groups remained responsible for care of the poor and ill and led in the development of early hospitals.

Major changes occurred during the Renaissance (1500–1700 AD) throughout Europe. Books became more available to universities, Da Vinci made his anatomical drawings, Leewenhoek invented the microscope, and medical, pharmacy and nursing schools were established.

During the Reformation, the British Parliament attempted to suppress the influence of the church through dissolution of monasteries and hospitals run by the church. As a result, "low" women took over the care of the sick in hospitals, bringing a dark period of history for health care. It was at this time that care of the poor became a societal rather than a religious responsibility. The English Poor Law of 1601 explicated how this would be done. If possible, parents, grandparents and children of "every poor, old, blind, lame, and impotent person or other person not able to work" were required to support such relatives. An overseer set able-bodied paupers to work and provided relief for those without relatives and unable to work. This system of "relief" was brought to New England by the colonists.

In America, some paupers were auctioned off to families either for care or work. This inhumane practice declined after the revolution and was replaced by contracting with one person to care for all the poor in one town. Because these privately owned almshouses made a profit (usually from the work of the "inmates," as they were known), towns frequently decided to run their own almshouses, which were sometimes called poorhouses, poor farms or work houses. Poverty and illness were viewed as signs of a character defect, moral weakness or punishment for sin. Therefore, some minimal gratitude for care was expected. Inmates were thus expected to contribute to their keep through work. Quarters were spartan and were expected to cost as little as possible. Privileges for leaving the premises were directly related to "good" behavior and the number of years of residence in a particular area.

During the early 1900s, privately owned "boarding homes" became available to the more affluent aged, and church-sponsored homes for the aged emerged. A certain number of deserving citizens who had fallen on hard times were often allowed to "spend their last days" at many of these homes through the donations of benefactors. A few institutions introduced a nurse to care for the bodily needs of those who required it, but only personal and custodial care were envisioned.

At the same time, able bodied workers were drawn from the poor houses. Convicts were sent to prisons. Orphanages were built to prevent exploitation of children without parents. Hospitals were established for the mentally ill and mentally retarded. Special homes were built for the blind and the deaf. Gradually, the other poor were differentiated, but the aged remained.

When the first Social Security Act was passed in 1935, conditions in county poor farms had become deplorable. The Act specifically denied anyone living in a public institution from receiving assistance payments. While the intent of this regulation was to force closure of county poor houses, it did not work out that way in many instances. Some counties leased the poor farm to a private individual, thus, it was no longer a public institution technically, so inmates could stay and still receive their payments. Residents who feared they could not find a better situation stayed where they were, but others left and found a private boarding house. Indeed, this exit to the community enabled some owners of large homes to maintain them by taking in "paid guests" during the depression, and ultimately gave impetus to the start of many proprietary homes.

Throughout the next thirty years, the number of aged continued to increase and homes for the aged became nursing homes increasing from 1270 in 1929, 7000 in 1954, 11,981 in 1965 to about 23,000 in 1980. During this period, hospitals became technologically more sophisticated, medical and hospital insurance became available to the majority of people, education of health professionals became more complex and new health professions emerged. Prior to 1965, there was little or no relationship between hospitals and nursing homes. Hospitals had grown out of the medical sciences and health care; nursing homes had grown from the welfare system and various private housing arrangements. Their missions differed, and their historical roots were not the same.

Hospitals and nursing homes were barely on speaking terms in 1965 when Congress passed Medicare and Medicaid which were enacted because of the need for improved health care of the elderly. This legislation has had both positive and negative effects on the aged and residents of nursing homes. The positive effects include (1) improved medical care for the elderly, both outpatient care and hospitalization; (2) mandated working relationships between hospitals and nursing homes; and (3) improved medical supervision and therapies for nursing home residents. It has also had several detrimental effects. First, the concept of "extended care" actually meant time-limited, post-hospital treatment as opposed to continued care of the physically and mentally impaired aged. This was a great disappointment to many people. Secondly, the legislation was based on the hospital/medical model which emphasizes disease rather than functional competence, treatment rather than quality of living and regulation of residents as a group rather than consideration of individuals. Third, and perhaps the greatest problem, was the emphasis on physical rather than emotional and mental needs.

Older Americans in the United States numbered 28 million in 1984, up from 3.1 million in 1900. During this same time period, the 65+ age group increased from 4 percent to 11.9 percent of the total population with a corresponding increase in life expectancy at birth from 48 to 74.7 years of age.

The more startling demographic shift, however, is occurring in the 85+ age group which now numbers 2.7 million people, a growth of 21-fold since 1900. By the year 2000 this group will be in excess of 4 million, more than the 65+ population of 1900!

These dramatic population shifts represent changes in the elderly themselves. The aging process is being delayed, as evidenced by the increasingly later onset of chronic diseases and the radical age increase of newly admitted nursing home residents from a mean age of 70 in 1970 to age 82 in 1982. These differences are attributed to the fact that each new cohort of elderly is better educated, more affluent, healthier, and more active than the previous cohort.

Because of the staggering implications of our changing societal composition, federal and state governments are making every effort to contain the growth and cost of publicly supported health care. As a result, all sectors of long term care, from housing to Alzheimer's care, have experienced a major shift in degree of illness of their clients as indicated by the following:

Housing (private and public)—residents are allowed to remain with support services if the person is in no danger to self or others.

Board and Care—residents look much like residents of Intermediate Care facilities a few years ago.

Intermediate Care (ICF)—residents look much like residents in skilled nursing facilities a few years ago.

Skilled Nursing (SNF)—residents look much like patients in hospitals a few years ago.

Hospitals—with a Prospective Payment System for Medicare patients, HMO's, ambulatory care centers and a greater emphasis on home health care, patients are leaving earlier and sicker, and often to nursing homes.

As the twentieth century ends, our traditional expectations from each sector changes. Hospitals are entering the nursing home business, nursing homes are becoming convalescent hospitals, and residential facilities are entering health care. Reassessment of missions and competition increase opportunities for creativity, leaving the aged themselves a bit confused but with many new choices.

PROFESSIONAL KNOWLEDGE AND
ADMINISTRATOR LICENSURE

The previous sections describe how long-term care organizations have evolved from almshouses, county poor farms, homes for the friendless and a host of small, religious, secular and charitable living arrangements. Their goal was to meet survival needs and little else. Superintendents of such facilities were either self-appointed or selected because of their ability to farm, nurse, administer "justice" or prepare inmates to "meet their maker." If he or she kept the place marginally clean, kept expenses down and did not allow any untoward incidents, nothing more was expected. Paid little, some were humane while others were not. Housekeeping, cooking, maintenance and other work was done by inmates so little staff was necessary. Professional staff was unheard of with the exception of an occasional nurse who (at best) had served a hospital apprenticeship or a clergyman to pastor their souls.

In 1903 when the word "gerontology" first appeared in the **Oxford English Dictionary,** it said, "see thanatology." It was not until 1945 that "gerontology" was even defined in Webster's dictionary. Gerontological knowledge and research were unheard of. There was no established body of knowledge available to persons working with the elderly. Knowledge of practitioners was no different than that of the general public. Therefore, intuition and common sense were the highest qualifications available in any organization.

Because knowledge and research in the field of aging is so recent, it explains (at least in part) today's wide gap between practice in the care of the elderly and available knowledge. There are very few long-time, knowledgeable practitioners in the field of aging. Few physicians have been educated in geriatric medicine even today. The same can be said of nurses. In 1976 only 9 percent of all schools of nursing required a course in geriatric nursing. While both medical and nursing students have experience working with the hospitalized elderly during training, far too few actually learn how to assess and care for the complex relationship of physiologic, psychosocial, nutritional and environmental problems. Education of social workers, physical therapists, recreational therapists and other professionals frequently have similar deficits. Most skilled health care professionals in the field of geriatrics are knowledgeable because personal interest and curiosity drives them to study available research and literature and to seek special educational programs.

There are, of course, other problems. Some people are more motivated by curing than by effecting gradual improvement or small but vital increments in function to improve quality of life. Others are uncomfortable with physical disability, mental confusion and the prospect of death. In addition, the public, families and many health care workers tend to attribute disabilities and behaviors of the elderly to the "aging process" rather than to physical disease, emotional problems, depression, nutrition or the environment. The result is most unfortunate, as many problems of the elderly go untreated, both in the community and in institutions.

Long-term care administrators have had similar problems related to education. Prior to the 1970s, only a handful of colleges or universities provided any educational programming for nursing home administrators. These programs were scattered across the United States and were unavailable to the vast majority of persons in the field. As a result, nursing home administrators had to rely upon themselves (personal experience, trial and error, commitment and intuition) and occasional educational meetings of trade or professional associations.

When licensure of nursing home administrators was federally mandated in 1971, it was very difficult to implement the recommended educational requirements for a variety of reasons. First, few higher educational institutions had monies to develop an entirely new curriculum. Few faculty persons had the time or knowledge to search the literature and select appropriate content from such diverse fields as psychology, medicine, gerontology, business, architecture, etc. Second, practicing administrators did not initiate this law. Indeed, this law was unique in three ways: (1) it was the first and (to date) only **federally** mandated health occupation licensure law; (2) because it evolved from external pressure to upgrade nursing homes receiving federal dollars, it had little support from practitioners in the field; and (3) it had no grandfather clause to accommodate established practitioners—all practitioners were required to take an examination after completing a specified number of class hours of education.

While licensure was federally mandated, each state was allowed to develop its own licensure law. As a result, nursing home administrator licensure laws differ greatly among the states. Some require minimal education beyond high school; some require a baccalaureate degree. This, of course, makes reciprocity for licensure among states very difficult and sometimes impossible. Not only does the amount of formal education vary, but the knowledge and skills of preceptors for internships (three to twelve months long) are diverse. This results in kaleido-scopic beliefs, knowledge and skills even among new administrators and a great variance in norms for practice. The latter is further intensified by the perspective of each administrator's previous work experience, such as hospital administration, mortuary science, public school teaching, social work, the ministry, accounting, pharmacy, business, nursing and many blue collar and white collar occupations.

Annual continuing education requirements for licensure are not stan-dard among states either. While continuing education is crucial for keeping administrators abreast of new laws and providing opportunities to share ideas, it is usually not possible to provide depth of content for individual learning needs.

Today, very few long-term care administrators have been educated in their field of practice, and most were educated **after** they entered the field, a direct reversal of practice in almost every established profession. Some observers have noted that the consequence has been a "show and tell" quality to professional education because there was no other way of passing on long-term care administrative practice. Until very recently, most new entrants to the field of nursing home administration have had no way of distinguishing untested, personal opinion from thoughtful analysis of tested knowledge in the long-term care setting.

The limited knowledge in this field has made it particularly vulnerable to outside criticism. Today, however, new knowledge from research in many disciplines seems to be emerging almost daily. Educational pro-grams for long-term care administrators are currently based on selected content from gerontology, business, hospital administration, and other fields. Greater testing of the applicability of these disciplines and expo-sure to other sciences related to the special problems of long-term care is generating new knowledge that will further delineate the field. Today's administrators are beginning to have resources that can help them to take new initiatives that will change the image of a nursing home by changing the home. The administrative challenge is to develop a truly therapeutic care environment with emphasis on quality of life, deter-mined individually with and for residents.

A LOOK TO THE FUTURE

This brief history of care of the poor, the aged and nursing home residents provides insight into the origins of institutional practices and public attitudes that are widely exhibited even today. Long-term care personnel need to reflect upon this past in order to understand their work environment as well as their own attitudes and practices. Such a perspective on history will help them to be less defensive about their work and to see the present as a stage in time rather than a constant.

The superintendent of a county poor farm was basically helpless because of societal attitudes and lack of resources; the administrator of a nursing home in the 1980s has the possibility of an exciting future. Educational programs for health care professionals are just beginning to turn their attention to the aging clientele. Research is starting to sort out opinions from facts. Sheer numbers of aged are forcing both personal and public attention to the aged. At no time in its history have there been greater resources, greater opportunities for learning and more room for the contribution of knowledgeable leaders.

REFERENCES

Dolan, Josephine. *History of Nursing,* Philadelphia, W. B. Saunders Co., 1968.

Hammerman, J., Friedsam, H. and Shore, H. Management Perspectives in Long Term Care Facilities, in Sherwood, Sylvia, Ed., *Long Term Care: A Handbook for Researchers, Planners, and Providers,* New York, Spectrum Publications, Inc., 1975.

McClure, Ethel. *More Than a Roof,* St. Paul, MN, Minnesota Historical Society, 1968.

Shore, Herbert. *History of Education for Long Term Care Administration,* paper presented at Faculty Institute LTC Administration, AUPHA, New Orleans, February 6, 1977.

Chapter 2

CHARACTERISTICS OF THE RESIDENTIAL CARE MODEL

RUTH STRYKER

In 1965 Medicare and Medicaid legislation thrust nursing homes from the welfare system into the health care system quite unwillingly. Concern about the quality of health care of elderly persons suggested that nursing homes should become more hospital-like. The concern was justified, but the remedy was based on a lack of understanding of the nature of chronic care compared to acute care. Even today, many policy-makers, boards, owners, administrators, and health care professionals are unable to articulate the major components of long-term care. Health care professionals have had predominantly acute care and hospital-based educations, and they bring practices and attitudes to elderly patients that are often counterproductive.

During the late 1980's, increased life expectancy, improved health habits, delayed onset of chronic disease, greater use of home health care and a host of supportive housing arrangements for the elderly, created new reasons for avoiding the medical model. To understand this view, it will be helpful to identify the major features of currently existing care models.

The medical/hospital model is 1) driven by high technology, 2) physician directed and 3) designed for persons with immediate acute health care needs. Treatment of disease is the principal goal. The nursing home/social model is 1) driven by basic principles of the psychosocial disciplines, 2) interdisciplinary team directed, and 3) designed for persons with chronic long-term physical and mental functional deficits. Quality of life is the major goal. The hospitality/hotel model is 1) driven by marketing data of client desires and satisfactions, 2) client directed, and 3) designed for persons with personal care needs. Security and comfortable living arrangements are major goals.

It is clear that as a person becomes less competent by virtue of disease, there is a loss of self-control which requires an increasing number of health and support services. However, the individual's sense of self-direction and self-esteem must be protected throughout these transitions. This can be accomplished through the development of the residential model.

The residential model integrates certain qualities of all three models. Health care must be delivered, but it is delivered in a residential setting which incorporates client driven decision making as much as possible in order to maintain the highest possible psychological and physical functioning. What is done for acute conditions in temporary settings is not appropriate for what is done for chronic conditions in long term settings. Provision of health care, attention to a quality living environment, and as much client decision making as possible characterize the residential model.

MAJOR AREAS OF EMPHASIS

SCIENTIFIC KNOWLEDGE: Hospital care is heavily rooted in biomedical and technological sciences while long-term care is more heavily rooted in the psychosocial sciences. The major problems of hospital patients are physical, while the major problems of older persons are social, economic, and emotional. The physical problems of the frail elderly are usually chronic, long-standing and under medical control. The nursing home deals with the more severe affective, cognitive, social and mental disorders. Supervised or supportive housing deals with similar but less severe psychological problems accompanied by less severe physical problems.

GOALS OF CARE: The main purpose of a hospital is to diagnose, treat and discharge its patients as quickly and efficiently as possible. The main purpose of a long-term care organization is to provide a secure psychosocial environment that promotes the highest physical and mental function for an improved quality of life. Rehabilitation and maintenance of physical and mental function must, of course, go hand in hand to accomplish this goal, but it is provided in a residential setting. In essence, the primary objective of a hospital is to provide a treatment environment; the primary objective of a nursing home is to provide maintenance and rehabilitation in a psychosocially health living environment. Health care is less intensive in the hospitality model which has a greater emphasis on personal care services (cleaning, nutrition, shopping, etc.).

DIAGNOSIS/CLIENT PROBLEM. A patient usually comes to a hospital with a primary physical diagnosis or complaint and organizational energies are focused on that primary problem. The long-term care client is far more complex. He or she has two or more chronic diseases, which may be fairly well controlled and of long duration, a variety of sensory deficits such as diminished hearing, vision and tactile sense, age-related conditions such as loss of stamina and energy, loss of mobility caused by stiff and aching muscles, and a host of psychological and mental conditions. In addition, there may be depression over loss of friends, spouse, children, home and diminished income. Even with loss of memory and confusion, an overlying depression can exacerbate mental symptoms.

All too frequently a depression goes untreated and can even be increased by living in an emotionally sterile or insensitive environment. Because the aged person lives in a long-term care organization with multiple chronic physical diseases, sensory losses, age-related symptoms and behavioral problems, a medical diagnosis has limited value in planning care. Therefore, functional diagnoses become mandatory. Knowing that an elderly person has arthritis gives guidance for directing treatment goals, but it tells nothing about needed support services. Data on medical diagnoses of nursing home residents rarely provide any clear picture of the multiplicity and complexity of actual problems or needs that confront personnel. Functional assessment is equally important for those who live in the hospitality model.

THERAPEUTIC EXPECTATIONS. For most hospital patients, the aim is to cure a disease or at least return home and resume normal activity. For most long-term care residents, however, there are few specific therapeutic aims except for goals in physical function. This can be replaced by more scientifically based programs and services that attempt to control or reduce the mental and physical effects of aging, to improve or at least maintain function and to enrich life at home or in a nursing home when discharge is not a truly viable option.

It is this author's contention that an unknown number of elderly can improve and live at a lesser level of care if this objective is taken more seriously by physicians and personnel in all types of health care organizations. Whether an aged person remains at home with depression from feeling like a burden to family over a period of time or enters an institutional environment devoid of social, intellectual, physical or other appropriate stimulation, the effect is the same; namely, the aged person is deprived of assessment and therapy. Lack of goals and expectations by health care professionals compound the aged person's sense of helplessness and hopelessness.

Most hospital patients and staff expect a positive outcome. Most long-term care patients, however, expect a negative outcome. This can become a self-fulfilling prophesy. When patients, families, physicians and staff think everything is "downhill from here on," nothing is done to try to make it otherwise. Fortunately for those who live in nursing homes where staff know better, quality of life is enhanced physically, socially, emotionally and mentally even when discharge is inadvisable. This, of course, includes terminally ill residents whose environment encompasses some of the qualities of the hospice movement as described in Chapter 22.

THE CLIENT'S ROLE. The hospital patient's role is to submit to appropriate care. Temporarily, this includes permitting dependence and giving up a certain degree of personal freedom in order to obtain appropriate outcomes. The long-term client's role is to participate in his or her own care, maintain individuality, live close to prized belongings, make choices about the daily routine, activities, their timing and to reject any activities that might increase dependence. However, if a frail elderly person is expected to take on the more traditional dependent role of a hospital patient, self-esteem is lowered and functional abilities are reduced. While temporary dependence can help to achieve positive therapeutic outcomes in acute care, long-term dependence results in a decision-free environment.

THE CARE GIVER' ROLE. The hospital care giver's role is clearly to direct and give care. The long-term care giver's role has not been so clearly defined. However, staff surely must (1) encourage self-direction, (2) create a flexible environment, (3) promote choices, (4) be a friend to clients, (5) help persons to help themselves in order to improve self-esteem and competency, (6) encourage individuality, (7) allow emotional expression, (8) promote affectional ties, and (9) support the family, or in some instances, serve as surrogate families. In other words, expediting care rather than giving care, a basic rehabilitation philosophy, needs to be developed in residential care settings.

This requires professional staff to give up some of their control in order to give residents more control over their lives. This requires a breakdown of the staff-resident caste line (Bowker). Betty Chang's study of situational factors affecting morale of institutionalized aged showed that resident control of daily activities was the strongest contributor to morale. In Tobin and Leiberman's research, passivity was found to be the only predictor of morbidity and mortality among persons going to nursing homes. They identified a heightened sense of mastery for residents as a key issue for long-term care staff. This requires an understanding that reduced control creates a sense of anonymity, lowers self-esteem, and produces apathy, a sense of powerlessness, and increased helplessness. In practice, this requires developing a tolerance for individual decision-making even if it is not thought to be "good" for the individual. Residents had rights prior to admission, and they need to have as many as possible after admission. Chapters 3 and 8 deal with many of these concerns in greater detail.

CARE SYSTEM. The hospital has basically a closed system for patients. Most major decisions are made by the physician from the decision to admit to the day of discharge. Other disciplines support and contribute to that care throughout the stay. Long-term care, however, is basically a more open system because there is a greatly altered distribution of power in decisions about care. First of all, residents have a greater "say." Nurses, social workers, families, administrators and other therapists have far broader decision-making authority and initiatives about care and services including opening the resident's life to the community. Their combined power and influence on care and outcomes is much greater than in a hospital. Even entry to the system differs. While the physician must approve a residential care admission, it is the family and resident who decide institutionalization is required, select a long-term care facility and arrange for admission, usually working with a social worker and nurse. The hospitality model is of course completely open to client decisions.

MEDICAL STAFF. In a hospital, there is an organized medical staff that is influential by virtue of their acknowledged expertise. They visit and monitor hospital care daily. This is not necessary in long-term care. Physicians usually see their patients once a month and work indirectly with a team of other persons who work directly with needs that are not in the physician's province of expertise. Physicians usually desire less input and are not organized as a staff, especially if they have little training or special interest in geriatric care. The multiplicity of problems of the aged requires a greater sharing of expertise with other persons and professions than in a hospital. In all models, it is critical that a full medical evaluation be done.

NURSING STAFF. A hospital staff is comprised of about three professional staff to one non-professional staff. For the most part, staff are educated in acute care and feel confident in their ability to deliver the care that is expected of them. Long-term care organizations have about one-third fewer staff per bed and have a ratio of three non-professionals to one professional staff person. Therefore, nurses (often without a geriatric background) must supervise a greater number of non-professionals, and they have fewer peers and other support people to call upon. The combination of greater responsibility, fewer professional back-up persons and less education in their field of practice presents formidable challenges for the professional nurse. This is as true for home care as it is for institutional care.

FAMILY IMPACT. The impact of families on the care of hospital patients is quite minimal. Their role is to receive medical and other information about their relative and to support the patient. In the residential setting, however, the family is very much involved in several aspects. First, the family initially selects the nursing home in most instances. After admission, they can become a very important part of the treatment system by providing information, some direct care and access to the external environment, other family members and the community. Family participation also requires some relinquishing of authority by personnel. Finally, families often need to receive care to deal with their grief, guilt, anger, and depression. Family services, dealt with in Chapter 16, require special personnel, knowledge and skills. In the home or hospitality setting, families provide many support services.

RESIDENT IMPACT. The social and psychological impact of the patient on organizational function is usually minimal or occasional in the hospital. In the residential or long-term care setting, however, the resident greatly influences (for better or worse) the behavior of other residents, staff and the general operation of programs and services. Encouraging greater control by residents is crucial. However, like any community, a wide variety of behaviors will be exhibited, and individualized interventions may be necessary when disruptive behavior occurs. The housing manager will find this a frequent area of concern and responsibility.

ARCHITECTURAL DESIGN. Hospitals are designed around the provision of services and the most efficient and cost effective use of personnel in delivering those services. Long-term care residential organizations should be designed around the concept of living and function of residents. Private accomodations are strongly recommended. However, if a double room is designed, a toe-to-toe bed arrangement rather than side-to-side beds provide both residents with greater privacy as well as a window. Furniture can be arranged in a manner that suggests more of a bed-living room rather than merely a bedroom.

Color can increase or decrease confusion as can the amount of glare or dark areas from lighting in halls, living rooms, activity rooms and dining rooms as described in Chapter 18. There are a host of other considerations that can improve self-esteem through greater independence such as the shape of door knobs, grab bars, the type of window openers, and the height of clothes poles in closets. Non-room space in long-term care organizations is not used for x-ray, lab, O.R., etc.; it is used for living space, privacy space, reading areas, conversation areas, social space, activities, etc.—features of a residence.

COST/REIMBURSEMENT. The per diem rate of hospitals is four to five times that of nursing homes. Indeed motel rates are often double that of nursing homes. Some observers think that nursing home care is our best health care bargain. However, because of the obvious difference in length of stay, nursing home care becomes very expensive for an individual over a prolonged time.

Payment of services for hospital care comes largely from insurance companies and Medicare while the payment of services for nursing home care comes mainly from private funds or Medicaid. Although long-term care insurance availability is growing rapidly, it is owned by few, so the impact on private resources can still overwhelm an individual or family. Home care and hotel models save both public and private dollars when intensive health needs are unnecessary.

ORGANIZATIONAL SUCCESS. The hospital can be considered an organizational success because its purpose (to diagnose, treat and discharge) is in agreement with the goals of its clients, staff, services and mission statement. Professional staff have been educated in their area of practice. While conflicts may arise about individual situations, they rarely relate to overall purpose and goals. Long-term care residential organizations, on the other hand, often exhibit many contradictions within themselves. Stated goals often conflict with actual care. Because of lack of education in geriatrics, physicians may withdraw from residents, and nurses may emphasize physical care without equal emphasis on rehabilitative and psychosocial care.

Most elderly, even those in board and care and skilled nursing homes, consider themselves well, but health care givers perceive them as ill. In addition, families are likely to expect dependence-oriented care. Apathy on the part of the public, a sense of hopelessness on the part of families, residents and other professionals and certain regulatory policies contribute to a state of mixed perceptions and expectations in many residential care settings. As a result, success is often defined quite differently by each party involved.

ADMINISTRATIVE DIRECTIONS

How do all of these factors influence the knowledge and performance skills needed by the administrator of a residential care organization? First of all, the administrator must take leadership in formulating a mission statement. A mission statement needs to include a commitment to education and research as well as care. It might include a specific target population, the Lutheran, Catholic or community elderly, or the elderly with particular disabilities, either mental or physical. The creative geriatric center provides parallel services, medical and social care. Seven major components can be identified: (1) medical care, (2) residential and personal care, (3) mental health care, (4) dying care, (5) education programs, (6) research activities and (7) community services. The administrator must also take leadership in educating the board and/or owners of what the real mission and potential accomplishments of the organization can be. Board members or owners must be committed to exploring creative efforts if the organization is to become a dynamic community resource.

Second, the administrator of a residential care organization must have some gerontological knowledge in order to take leadership in the quality of care through environmental intervention. When a hospital administrator resigns, the quality of direct care is not likely to be influenced. However, when an administrator of a long-term care organization leaves, the entire atmosphere of the organization may quickly alter from a therapeutic environment to one that is not or vice versa. The quality of care is dependent upon the quality of the psychosocial environment set by the administrator.

A second reason for gerontological knowledge relates to the physical design and interior of the building, because it must be planned with knowledge of sensory changes, physical adaptive needs and mental states that are found in many residents. The administrator must also understand that self-esteem and morale of residents is nourished by the attitudes and general atmosphere of the organization. Clinical knowledge helps to identify which routines, procedures, policies and organizational practices diminish life satisfaction of residents. The employer must have a clear idea of what personal characteristics employees need if they are to enhance residents' quality of life. In summary, this knowledge provides a base for selecting appropriate programs, personnel services, architectural design, interior decoration and even furniture, all of which can make the difference between dependence and independence, self-esteem and depression, or satisfaction and despair.

Third, the administrator must have broad and diverse management and interpersonal skills that allow him or her to function with fewer professionals, in an environment with conflicting and sometimes indifferent participants, with fewer trained assistants and department heads, and a somewhat hostile public environment. Most hospitals have a pyramidal organizational structure with several levels of middle management, many with special expertise to support financial, personnel, and planning decisions. By contrast, long-term residential care organizations have a flat structure with few if any middle management positions. These factors, of course, place a wider variety of responsibilities on the administrator. As a result, the administrator must assume yet another role, that of educator. Staff development, in fact, may become a primary role in many instances.

Finally, in order to be successful in administering services to the elderly, a more than superficial knowledge of change theory is required to lead an organization from the hospital model to a therapeutic residential model that constantly asks itself, "Would I like to live here?" John Gardner states in his book, **Self-Renewal,** "Knowledge will be a safe weapon only if it is linked to a deeply rooted conviction that organizations are made for men and not men for organizations. The whole purpose of such knowledge is to design environments conducive to individual fulfillment. . . . " Succeeding chapters will suggest ways of accomplishing this.

REFERENCES

Bowker, Lee H. *Humanizing Institutions for the Aged.* Lexington, MA, Lexington Books, 1982.

Chang, B. "Focus of Control, Trust, Situational Control and Morale of the Elderly" *International Journal of Nursing Studies.* 16: 169–181, 1979.

Gardner, John. *Self-Renewal.* New York, Harper and Row, 1963.

Harel, Z. and L. Noelker. "Social Integration, Health and Choice. Their Impact on the Well-Being of Institutionalized Aged." *Research on Aging,* 4: 97–111, 1982.

Tobin, Sheldon and Leiberman, Morton. *Last Home for the Aged.* San Francisco, CA, Jossey-Bass, 1976.

Chapter 3

WORKER MOTIVATIONS, ATTITUDES AND PERCEPTIONS

GEORGE KENNETH GORDON

INTRODUCTION

A nursing home does not function in a vacuum. It is, in sociological terms, a social institution; the way the nursing home works on a day-to-day basis is a reflection of the beliefs of the local community as well as the larger society in which the home exists. These beliefs are especially expressed in the interchange among the staff, the residents, and residents' families. How this interplay of beliefs is meshed or mismatched has important implications for the outcomes of the care provided. This is a difficult area of inquiry. Nevertheless, the consequences of the way these beliefs interface and are expressed in the daily round of activity in the nursing home are so important that prudent managers cannot afford to ignore them.

The term "beliefs" has been introduced above as a very general term. What follows is an attempt to examine four specific areas in which beliefs are involved—work motivation, staff attitudes, public opinion, and perceptions. These are all areas which not only can be scrutinized and monitored by managers but also can be influenced by managers with important implications for the way the organization functions and its outcomes.

A FRAME OF REFERENCE

In their book, **The Art of Japanese Management**, Pascale and Athos state that American managers tend to be preoccupied with strategy, structure, and system. They go on to contend that this preoccupation can produce organizations which are arid wastelands, which reduce the people who do the work of the organizations to cogs which are required to respond mechanically to changes in strategy, structure, and system. They present an unpleasant picture of the organization as an inhumane machine in which the demands of strategy, structure, and system wear away at each other and grind each other down.

These authors do not in any way denigrate the importance of strategy, structure, and systems as primary management responsibilities. Indeed, they are quite explicit in expressing their admiration for the excellence with which certain organizations fine-tune these three management functions.

They contend, however, that there are other elements of managerial function that must be tended to in order to convert strategy, structure, and system into bottom-line outcomes. There can be no outcomes, in fact, apart from people to enact them. Strategies, structures, and systems are nothing more than pure abstractions until real flesh and blood people accept them, or claim ownership of them, and enact them into performance and accomplishment, i.e. the bottom line.

Pascale and Athos thus present a challenging question: what does it take to develop and cultivate a lively organization which can attain a high level of effectiveness across time? They present the suggestion that it is entirely possible to design an elegant, parsimonious, and thoroughly rational organization, which simply will not work.

What Pascale and Athos say is perhaps illustrated by the Hamm's beer advertising campaign of a few years back which featured a woodsman and a grizzly bear. For years, the Hamm's beer commercials had featured an animated cartoon presentation of a bear who encountered "the Perils of Pauline" in segment after segment on behalf of Hamm's beer sales. The woodsman and the bear, however, were not animated cartoon presentations. They presented a real man and a real bear doing very ordinary things together.

Viewers were enthralled. The woodsman and his bear gained the status of celebrity and had a nationwide following of admirers.

In their swing on the celebrity circuit, the woodsman (really, the bear's trainer) was frequently asked how he got the bear to do the things the bear did in the commercials. His stock answer to this question was, "I never ask the bear to do anything that will embarrass him."

In essence, the trainer was saying that if you want to work with a bear (a wild animal that has never adapted to domestication), you had better start by understanding the nature of the bear. And you never ask the bear to do something which contradicts or violates the bear's fundamental nature. If you do, you run the risk of reducing the bear to a caricature of itself, on the one hand, or of provoking the bear's active resistance and hostility on the other hand.

Probably the charm of the Hamm's beer commercials was that the bear conveyed a sense of great dignity in performing his part in the commercials. The bear was not degraded or reduced to a caricature of what a bear should be nor was he provoked into expressions of rage and resistance under coercion.

There is an important point here with respect to organizational management. Simply put, it is entirely possible for managers to design elegant and rational systems, structures, and strategies for organizational performance which are not acceptable to the people who must implement them. If it is organizational performance that you are concerned about, you had better take time to consider the requirements of the people who must accomplish the performance — and "never ask the bear to do anything that will embarrass him."

This point is not to be taken lightly. There are, in fact, specific cases to illustrate the point, and perhaps none are more pointed than the mechanization of coal mining in Great Britain following World War II.

There can be no doubt that the mechanization of coal mining was a great boone to the miners. It relieved them of the tedious and back-breaking labor of cutting the coal by hand with a pick-ax and then loading the cut coal by hand into a hutch. Mechanization obviously made the work much easier.

Surprisingly, however, grievances and work disruptions increased with the introduction of mechanization and productivity suffered. It simply did not make sense.

It did not make sense, that is, until management discovered that a persistent fear in the back of every miner's mind was the fear of being caught, alone, isolated in an underground disaster.

Under the manual labor procedures through which mining had been carried on for 200 years, it was not likely that an individual miner would be caught as an isolated individual in event of a cave-in or explosion. Miners always worked together in cooperating groups.

Mechanization had the unwitting effect of isolating the miners from each other, each man efficiently operating a particular machine. Mechanization thus presented a thoroughly rational way of mining which was elegant and efficient as well as freeing the miners from the degradation of lying on their sides in seeping water in order to cut coal with a pick-ax from a seam of coal that might be only 18 inches high. But the mechanization also contradicted a very fundamental human value which was critically important to the miners as people.

The thoroughly elegant and efficient technical system of mechanized mining had to be adjusted and accommodated to the distinctly human needs of the people who implemented (and were among the major beneficiaries of) mechanized mining procedures. The potential excellence of the technical system had to accommodate to the psychosocial system of the miners.

What was at stake in the mechanization of British coal mining was the need for management to understand and accommodate the distinctly human needs and motivations of the miners. This is akin to what Pascale and Athos are driving at when they say that good management involves more than a preoccupation with strategies, structures, and systems. Management thinking must also account for the needs and motivations of the people who must do the day-today work of the organization.

WORK MOTIVATION

When we turn our thoughts to work motivations, there are two basic concepts that managers need to keep in mind:

1. The workers need to know that you care about them.
2. The workers need to be their own unique selves.

On first reading, these two propositions sound like they come directly from the humanistic psychology which was popular among many organizational consultants during the 60s and 70s. One observer has suggested that those human relations consultants played the role of court jesters to American corporations in those decades.

No such "straw-man," satirical, sarcastic, or cynical context should be attached to these propositions currently. These two propositions are set forward quite simply as guiding principles for what managers must do to develop organizations through which well-conceived strategies, systems, and structures can be implemented.

In very homely fashion, these two propositions define the difference between excellent and ordinary organizations. It is commitment and attention to these two propositions in excellent organizations that provide the lubricant that keeps strategies, stuctures, and systems from grinding each other away.

The innovative manager who aspires to excellence in organizational performance grasps these two fundamental propositions and translates them into action principles for the organization. This is the point at which formal theories become useful guides to action.

CARING

How, for example, does a nursing home organization express to its rank-and-file employees that the organization cares about them? Herzberg's two-factor theory of work motivation suggests that you express that you care about them by treating them well, that you treat them as best you possibly can by providing them a decent place to work.

According to Herzberg, that means that you provide the best possible work environment that you are capable of providing. Herzberg goes on to list the components or categories of consideration through which the management conveys to employees that the organization cares about them:

Wages
Benefits
Policies and Administration
Supervision
Human Relations
Security
Status

Herzberg contends that it is through the above that management expresses to nursing home employees that the organization cares about them. He is unrelenting on this point. Any toleration of less than the best possible conveys shabby treatment to rank and file employees; it says that the management does not really care about them.

Some managers may conceive "caring about the employees" in terms of being able to address each employee by name or maintaining a "tickler file" of birthdays and employment anniversaries which are to be acknowledged. Herzberg's list goes far beyond such techniques. A careful elaboration of what constitutes excellence in terms of each item in the above list will quickly reveal that the nursing home organization and its management must be both up-front and out-front in committing the resources of the organization and accepting responsibility for the pursuit of excellence. That is how the organization expresses caring for the rank and file employee.

Employees are not dumb. They may lack technical competence and precision in defining the constraints within which the nursing home must perform, but they are not dumb. Generally, they are forgiving with respect to external constraints on organizational operations but they have a fine sensitivity to the authenticity of a manager's commitment to excellence in providing a decent place to work. They know when management cares about them.

PERFORMANCE

The manager who is a student of formal work motivation theories will recognize, at this point, that Herzberg's itemization of how an organization expresses caring about employees only has to do with providing a decent place to work. It does not guarantee employee performance, i.e. the bottom line.

When we focus on performance, we get back to the analogy of the bear in the T.V. commercials. The trainer said that he never asked the bear to do anything that would embarrass the bear. He studied the nature of the bear and never asked the bear to do anything that contradicted or violated the nature of the bear. The result was that the bear performed with apparent dignity and ease.

Human beings are far more diverse, complex, and adaptable than bears. In this sense, it is better to forget about the bear. Human performance in the provision of nursing home care takes us to an entirely different plane of sophistication and values.

Nevertheless, the point is well taken. If it is performance in the delivery of nursing home services that you are concerned about, and you must manage the organization of the delivery of those services, you must take account of the nature of the people who deliver those services. Delivery of the services must include opportunity for the people providing the services to be their own unique selves. Provision of the services must fit the nature of the people providing the services in order for the people to perform with a sense of dignity and ease.

With respect to designing work so that people can be their own unique selves, Herzberg is helpful again. What he says is that you must design work so that you **use** people well. That means that the work must fit the capabilities of the people doing the work and provide appropriate opportunities to advance and refine those capabilities.

Earlier, Herzberg was quoted as saying that you express the fact that you care about employees by **treating** them well and that is a matter of providing a decent work environment. With respect to motivating employees for quality work performance, he says that you must use them well and that means designing jobs which provide opportunity for:

1. Achievement
2. Recognition for accomplishment
3. Challenging work
4. Increased responsibility
5. Growth and development

Herein lies a challenge to the creativity, problem solving, and moral commitment of nursing home administrators. A great deal of the day-to-day work of nursing home employees is repetitive and routinized. There is a challenge, therefore, in recruiting and selecting employees who will find challenge and opportunity for achievement in the provision of nursing home care. More important, there is the challenge of developing effective, multiple ways of providing recognition, of expanding work responsibilities for employees as they mature in their work capabilities, and of redesigning jobs and training programs so as to maintain appropriate growth and development for individual employees. The administrator needs to understand the employees and cultivate the options for growth and development in the work itself.

All of the foregoing brings us to a key question: what are the characteristics of nursing home employees that must be taken into account in the design and management of the work itself? What are the needs and requirements of the workers which the work must satisfy?

Generalizations are always risky because as soon as they are stated they are likely to generate thoughts and recollections of specific exceptions. With that limitation in mind, the following generalizations are presented for your consideration:

1. **They tend to be service oriented.** They are consciously committed to the belief that service to fellow human beings is a self-validating good which needs no further explanation or justification. Furthermore, they tend to believe that providing such service is legitimate work. They like to work with people and they get personal satisfaction out of helping others.
2. **They tend to be relations-motivated.** Such people believe that people are the most important things in the world, that organizations exist for people and not the other way around, and they place high value on being able to develop and maintain congenial and mutually supportive human relationships. They expect their work to

provide an arena in which their relationships-motivation can be expressed and satisfied.

3. **They have a need for recognition.** It is a secondary characteristic of relations-motivated people. When human relationships have been established, the need for recognition of quality performance becomes a pressing need.

This is especially true of nursing home personnel. Most of their work consists of providing personal care and services which are transient events in time leaving no concrete residual or artifact demonstrating the quality of the caring act or service. They need recognition from others, especially from coworkers and management, in order to sustain high quality work performance over time.

4. **They tend to be group-centered** with respect to the organization of work. They are not loners but prefer to work in stable interdependent teams with predictable and dependable coworkers.

5. **They increasingly see themselves as professionals.** The body of knowledge about nursing home residents and their care has mushroomed during the past decade. Consequently, many nursing home employees are aware that there are special skills and know-how in providing quality nursing home care. Not just anyone can do it. Nursing home personnel increasingly see themselves as having "careers" in long-term care, and career people are not simply job-holders. They have valued competencies to be nurtured and developed. How do organizational practices accommodate such employee perceptions and expectations?

6. **They are conflicted about their work.** Nursing homes are a fairly recent social innovation; there is widespread misunderstanding, confusion and controversy over the role and function of nursing homes in our society. For some people, nursing homes are a source of guilt and shame. There are, therefore, ample opportunities for nursing home personnel to encounter a sense of personal contradiction or conflict over their employment in the nursing home.

Organizational practices which stimulate or aggravate the sense of conflict or contradiction are debilitating to personnel performance. This is especially true with respect to how organizational policies and practices influence control versus independence of the residents (see Chapter 8).

These six characteristics of nursing home employees present a global description and they suggest the areas of concern that managers need to take into account in order to develop and maintain a motivating work environment. Managers who do not tend to these employee needs or who develop work systems and practices which subtly subvert the work requirements of personnel thereby undermine the potential for commitment and quality performance in the provision of care. The resultant discontent of employees (though they may not be able to define precisely the cause of discontent) will be expressed in poor work performance, high turnover, and a general sense of mediocrity communicated to residents, families, and the community at large.

THE EXTERNAL ENVIRONMENT

The matter of conflict, contradiction, and controversy over the public image and opinion of nursing homes is an area that deserves clarification. As indicated earlier, public controversy over nursing homes is a fact of life for the nursing home field. Moreover, nursing home personnel frequently express their dismay and sense of personal hurt because of across-the-board condemnations of nursing homes which are sometimes made by nursing home critics. This cannot but influence the way personnel feel about their employment in a nursing home—and the most committed personnel are likely to feel most disturbed.

It is important, therefore, for everyone connected with nursing homes to clarify the nature of the controversies wherever possible. The literature of the field includes multiple suggestions and explanations for the sources of the controversy and quite possibly all of them have some credibility and are worthy of scrutiny. One of the most provocative suggestions is that the controversy stems from deep-seated fear. An advocate of the "fear hypothesis" writes as follows:*

Antipathy toward nursing homes by the general public, potential employees, and potential clientele, as well as policymakers, stems from eight distinct sources. Several of these are more related to the job nursing homes are asked to do rather than the institutions themselves. They include:

1. Fear of one's own possible physical and/or mental deterioration which might cause loss of control of body and behavioral functions

---

*Ruth Stryker-Gordon, personal communication.

resulting in intolerable dependence or strain upon family members, strangers, or public dollars.

2. Fear that a family member will become so dependent and/or disruptive to other family members that outside services or institutional care will be required. This is a two-edged sword—the patient feels rejected by the family and the family feels guilty for being unable or unwilling to care for the person.

3. Fear that all nursing homes are like the worst portrayed in the media. While the purpose of such exposés is to close incompetent and unscrupulous homes, it creates a generalized suspicion of incompetence, lack of humanity, and lack of ethics in all nursing homes.

4. Fear that a prolonged period of physical or mental dependence will deplete either one's own financial resources or one's inheritance.

5. Fear that anger and guilt from present and/or past family relationships may result in inappropriate decisions for care.

6. Fear that knowledge needed for distinguishing between appropriate and inappropriate nursing homes is inadequate if one must be selected.

7. Fear of the unknown associated with any move to a new community, new job, or new role experienced by persons of all ages.

8. The sense of permanency associated with nursing home placement has a potential for drastically reducing an individual's sense of control and independence.

This "fear hypothesis," as elaborated by Stryker-Gordon, is very persuasive both in scope, explanatory power, and intuitive appeal for people who are well acquainted with nursing homes.

Several years ago, a graduate student in the School of Business at the University of Minnesota conducted a small marketing study which quite unintentionally produced a set of data which lends credence to the fear hypothesis. He surveyed a group of older adults living in a high-rise in Michigan. They responded very positively in their assessments of various aspects of the nursing homes they were acquainted with: cleanliness, quality of care, food services, staff attitudes, activities programs, etc. Nevertheless, when asked how they would feel if they were informed that they needed to be admitted to a nursing home the next day, the overwhelming response was the expression of depression, sadness, and despair. When asked to comment on the reasons for this response, the explanations had to do almost entirely with the loss of personal freedom. Summing up, the respondents had very few complaints about the way nursing homes perform their functions, but the prospect of personally requiring nursing home care was depressing and, perhaps, hateful. The study supports Stryker-Gordon's statement that some of the fear of nursing homes seems to relate to "the job nursing homes are asked to do rather than the institutions themselves."

The Michigan study described above was a limited, small scope, preliminary inquiry. Nevertheless, it is worthy of note because there is all but a total lack of systematic study of the public perceptions of nursing homes. This is most unfortunate because it leaves every citizen with the difficult task of making sense out of the tangle of rhetorical arguments about nursing homes encountered in the media and legislatures of our nation.

Not only nursing home employees, but the elderly themselves meet a host of contradictory behaviors wherever they go. Ageism, a prejudicial attitude toward the elderly, is an all too common social phenomenon manifested by discriminatory practices and bolstered by unsubstantiated stereotyping. Kastenbaum states that health professionals hold these same societal attitudes, resulting in a reluctance to work with the elderly. Indeed, even elderly persons sometimes have a gnawing sense of self-reproach that seems to stem from becoming what one once was prejudiced against. This is both insidious and elusive because the causes go unidentified and many false beliefs go unchallenged.

Studies of attitudes of health care professionals toward the elderly, while sometimes contradictory, indicate generally negative attitudes across professions. Physicians, nurses, social workers and dentists are of particular interest because they have so many elderly clients.

Palmore's **Facts on Aging Quiz** has been administered to thousands of health professionals. West and Levy surveyed 170 physicians across twenty-eight specialties in Texas. All age cohorts, except the 60–70 year olds, tended to be negatively biased. Most physician scores were no better than university undergraduate scores and those in practice areas most likely to treat the elderly did no better than those in pediatrics. On a more positive note, Green found third year medical students were quite positive about their feelings and contacts with old patients.

Michael Strayer's study found that over forty-five percent of Ohio dentists chose the elderly as their least preferred patients. The dentist's scores on the **Facts on Aging Quiz** were similar to those of the general population. However, dentists with the largest percentage of elderly patients and those who worked in nursing homes had the highest scores.

Wolk and Wolk's study of 220 social workers found that only twenty-five percent chose to work with the elderly. Among 4000 student nurses, the aged were identified as the least popular age group to work with (Feldbaum and Feldbaum).

Education, but not·experience, is a critical variable related to positive attitudes in many studies. The more educated social workers, nurses, supervisors in a nursing home, and home health care personnel had more positive attitudes than·less educated persons in similar positions (Kosberg, Cohen and Mendlovitz). Brower's study of Florida nurses found that the greater the contact with elderly persons, the greater the amount of negative stereotyping. Those with positive grandparent relationships tended to have more positive attitudes (Robb).

Administrator sensitivity to these issues and awareness of these findings should guide the selection, training, and evaluation of employees in any type of geriatric service or program. It is certainly critical to realize that mere exposure to the elderly is as likely to generate negative attitudes as positive ones.

A PERSPECTIVE ON PERCEPTIONS

Recently, a technology for measuring people's perceptions of nursing homes has been developed at the University of Minnesota. It involves an adaptation of procedures developed by Thomas Holmes and his colleagues for measuring the stressfulness of life change events. Specifically, the Minnesota adaptation involves the inclusion of the life event, "becoming a nursing home resident."

Years of study with the Holmes technology shows that people share a fundamental understanding of the relative stressfulness of the forty-three life change events that are included in the standard Holmes measuring instrument. The agreement is strong enough that Holmes has developed a set of standard life stress point weightings for each of the forty-three events as displayed in Table 3-1.

The Minnesota adaptation of the Holmes instrument is called the Nursing Home Perceptions Survey Instrument (NHPSI). The measuring qualities of the instrument and procedures for analyzing data gathered through the NHPSI have been explored over a period of eight years and the instrument has been demonstrated to be dependable and capable of producing data worthy of high levels of confidence.

What then do we know about the public image of nursing homes through the use of the NHPSI? First of all, it must be stated that the baseline data was gathered entirely in Minnesota and the bulk of the

TABLE 3-1

SOCIAL READJUSTMENT RATING SCALE

Rank	Life Event	Stress Point Value
1	Death of spouse	100
2	Divorce	73
3	Marital separation	65
4	Jail term	63
5	Death of close family member	63
6	Personal injury or illness	53
7	Marriage	50
8	Fired at work	47
9	Marital reconciliation	45
10	Retirement	45
11	Change in health of family member	44
12	Pregnancy	40
13	Sex difficulties	39
14	Gain of new family member	39
15	Business readjustment	39
16	Change in financial state	38
17	Death of close friend	37
18	Change to different line of work	36
19	Change in number of arguments with spouse	35
20	Mortgage over $10,000	31
21	Foreclosure of mortgage or loan	30
22	Change in responsibilities at work	29
23	Son or daughter leaving home	29
24	Trouble with in-laws	29
25	Outstanding personal achievement	28
26	Wife begin or stop work	26
27	Begin or end school	26
28	Change in living conditions	25
29	Revision of personal habits	24
30	Trouble with boss	23
31	Change in work hours or conditions	20
32	Change in residence	20
33	Change in schools	20
34	Change in recreation	19
35	Change in church activities	19
36	Change in social activities	18
37	Mortgage or loan less than $10,000	17
38	Change in sleeping habits	16
39	Change in number of family get-togethers	15
40	Change in eating habits	15
41	Vacation	13
42	Christmas	12
43	Minor violations of the law	11

data was gathered in the Minneapolis-St. Paul metropolitan area. Furthermore, the 1,100 respondents in the baseline study were health care personnel or people associated directly with a nursing home (including residents and their families).

Perhaps the most salient finding of the baseline study is that the 1,100 respondents produced an average of 62 life-stress points for the event, "becoming a nursing home resident." You can now examine the stress point values for the forty-three events listed in Table 3-I and make some observations. The baseline group perceived "becoming a nursing home resident" as being more stressful than getting married (50 points) or a personal injury or illness (53 points), about equally as stressful as the death of a close family member or a jail term (63 points), somewhat less stressful than a marital separation (65 points), and considerably less stressful than a divorce (73 points) or the death of a spouse (100 points). We now have a way for people to express their perceptions of nursing homes in a common frame of reference for interpretation.

Many colleagues who were involved in this research have been surprised at the score of 62 for "becoming a nursing home resident." They had expected the score to be much higher. When questioned as to why they expected higher scores, their answers usually referred to the way nursing homes are covered in the mass media.

A very important finding for nursing home personnel is the fact that there were very few extremely high scores. If individual scores in excess of 200 points are called high, then there were only thirteen high scores among the 1,100 people in the baseline group. In other words, slightly more than 1 percent of the baseline respondents attributed high life stress scores to "becoming a nursing home resident." In fact, there were not many individual scores in excess of 100 points. These findings should help nursing home personnel to evaluate the significance of extremely critical public statements about nursing homes.

There were seventy nursing home residents in the baseline group. These residents produced an average stress point score of 56 for "becoming a nursing home resident" as compared with 63 for nursing home employees and 65 for families of nursing home residents. Both families and nursing home personnel should find reassurance in these data; they indicate that the residents perceive the accommodation to nursing home living as a less stressful task than do either the employees or the residents' families.

The baseline data also show that stress scores are directly correlated with age. Young adults produce higher average scores (in the 70s and 80s) than do older adults whose scores range from low 50s and into the 60s. The importance of this finding lies in the fact that a substantial number of nursing home personnel are young women in the twenty- and thirty-year-old brackets. It is important for these younger employees to grasp the fact that they are likely to attribute far more stress to nursing home living than do older employees or the residents themselves. It is not a question of whose perception is "better," but rather the need for awareness and acceptance of differences of perceptions.

Finally, the baseline study suggests a need for all of us to find ways to minimize and ameliorate the stress incurred by a new resident in the transition to nursing home living. What do 62 additional stress points mean for the new resident?

Holmes and his associates have found through twenty-five years of research that when a person accumulates as many as 300 life stress points in one calendar year because of changes in that person's life, that individual is 80 percent predictable for the onset of serious illness. That is, people who have accumulated 300 life stress points in the course of one year are vulnerable and at risk—and as life stress totals rise beyond 300, so does the vulnerability and, consequently, morbidity and mortality rates.

Preliminary studies at the University of Minnesota suggest that the typical person presenting for admission to a nursing home has a previous twelve-month life change history totaling approximately 300 points. What are the consequences of taking on an additional 62 stress points for the transition to nursing home living? This question should give us pause to ponder what needs to be done to ease the transition. It may just be that well-conceived ameliorative efforts would have important implications for both the public image of nursing homes as well as the self-image of nursing home personnel, and most important of all, the well-being of the new nursing home resident.

In addition to the data from the baseline study, systematic surveys of the perceptions of the general citizenry have been conducted in five small towns in Minnesota, Wisconsin, Iowa, and Indiana. These studies indicate that NHPSI scores, in general, are five to ten points higher in these smaller communities than the scores associated with the baseline group. More important, however, are the distinctive differences among these five communities in terms of the NHPSI scores produced by the age/sex cohorts. Each community seemed to have its own "fingerprint" or "culture" of perceptions of nursing homes. There was a distinctive weave to the fabric of perceptions in each community.

These findings indicate that the nursing homes in each of these five communities function in subtly different environments. These differences also suggest distinctive strategies for the various nursing homes with respect to recruitment and selection of manpower, program development, public relations, and potential for influencing the public image of the nursing home in those communities. These, in turn, translate into ways of enhancing the motivations and satisfactions of nursing home personnel and the quality of services provided to the nursing home residents.

THE IMPACT OF BELIEFS ON HEALTH STATUS

Unfortunately, many treatment decisions for the elderly are made by persons who hold many of the beliefs described in the foregoing sections. Good intentions and kind impulses do not replace scientific inquiry about patients conditions and behavior. Persons working with the elderly must become acutely aware of their own attitudes and need to observe the effect of newly acquired behaviors have on their clients.

In addition, health care professionals need to learn how to 1) control underlying disease, 2) prevent further physical and emotional impairment (iatrogenic complications), 3) restore function whenever possible, and 4) modify the environment for maximum function. At least some myths lose their potency when knowledge is increased.

A few examples from those who know gerontological care will illustrate these points. Dr. Everett Smith from the University of Wisconsin reports that consistent mild exercise by 70 year-olds decreases blood pressure, increases cardiac output and increases muscle strength. In other words inactivity, not aging, causes many frailties, even in a nursing home. Nursing home residents who used wheelchairs, but did not have an identified reason for doing so, learned to walk when staff expectations and helping responses changed (McDonald). Rehabilitated stroke victims lost their independence and abilities when they were "taken care of" by family members both at home and in the nursing home setting (Anderson).

Sperbeck, postulating that we underestimate the role of environment, set about altering factors that produce institutional dependency. He reduced functional dependency of residents through staff training which included 1) more information about the aged, 2) encouraged staff to observe the influence of their actions and 3) taught operant behavior management. The time formerly used by staff to reinforce dependency was used to provide supportive care to increase independence.

There have been many studies of geriatric rehabilitation programs in a variety of settings—rehabilitation centers, hospitals, and nursing homes. The success rates are very high, ranging from 61 to 89 percent being discharged to the community (Kaplan & Ford, Reed & Gessner, and Wagner & Hilger). The cost of rehabilitation (average time about four weeks) is high, but it saves money after about six to twelve months because it prevents the cost of prolonged dependency.

Rubenstein et al attribute the positive results of an innovative geriatric assessment and treatment unit to several factors including staff expectations for improvement. They also concluded that the initial additional expenditure produced later benefits that increased patient function and lowered overall costs because long-term care in a dependent state was prevented.

CONCLUSION

This chapter began with the assertion that a nursing home is a social institution in which the conduct of day-to-day activities reflects the beliefs of the local community and the larger society in which the organization exists. This statement was based on what we know about employees, residents, and residents' families and the dynamics of what is known in the behavioral sciences as the self-fulfilling prophesy. That is, people act on what they believe and thereby what they believe is made manifest or enacted as documentable reality. This process plays itself out as a chicken-and-egg conundrum in which what people observe influences what they believe and what they believe influences the way they behave which, in turn, determines what falls within the domain of what they can possibly observe.

The self-fulfilling prophesy is sometimes identified as **the vicious cycle** or the **vicious circle**. These latter terms introduce a negative, pejorative connotation of relentless reiteration, recreation, and recycling of data confirming one's own cherished beliefs or worst suspicions (as the case may be) about the nature of reality. This is such a bleak picture as to be quite unacceptable for the long term care administrator.

It raises the spector of a mechanistic or deterministic world in which what will be will be and there is no use trying to change that reality. Such a viewpoint is all but totally incompatible with the concepts subsumed in terms such as management, administration, leadership, and creativity.

It might quite justifiably be said that the fundamental purpose of this book is to explore what can be done by enlightened, committed, creative, and competent long-term care administrators to break up and defeat the effects of the self-fulfilling prophesy. The chapters that follow are not of the cookbook, recipe, and prescription variety. They are intended to suggest what can be done by administrators who have been liberated to explore the possibilities of disciplined and creative combination and recombination of scientifically developed knowledge in pursuit of the highest ideals of quality of life for residents in long term-care facilities. The book is intended to be a catalyst for the reader encouraging her or him to venture into areas and possibilities which the authors of these chapters can hardly imagine.

REFERENCES

Anderson, E. Follow-up of Stroke Patients. Lecture. University of Minnesota, May, 1979.

Bowker, Lee. *Humanizing Institutions for the Aged.* Lexington, MA. Lexington Books, 1981.

Brower, T. "Social Organizations and Nurses' Attitudes Toward Older Persons." *Journal of Gerontological Nursing.* 11:1:17, 1981.

Cass, Eugene L. and Zimmer, Frederick G., (Eds.). *Man and Work in Society.* New York, Van Nostrand Reinhold, 1975, 313 pages.

Feldbaum E. and M. Feldbaum. "Caring for the Elderly: Who Dislikes it Least?" *Journal of Health Politics,* Policy and Law. 5:62–71, 1981.

Gordon, George K. "The Social Readjustment Value of Becoming a Nursing Home Resident." *The Gerontologist.* Vol. 25, No. 4, 1985.

Green, Susan et al. "Medical Student Attitudes Toward the Elderly". *Journal of American Geriatrics.* 31:5:305, May 1983.

Hersey, Paul and Blanchard, Kenneth H. *Management of Organizational Behavior.* Englewood Cliffs, N.J., Prentice Hall, 1982, 343 pages.

Herzberg, Frederick. One More Time: How Do You Motivate Employees? *Harvard Business Review.* January–February, 1968, pp. 53–62.

Holmes, Thomas H. and Rahe, Richard H. "The Social Readjustment Rating Scale. *Journal of Psychosomatic Research.* Volume 11, (1967), p. 213.

Kaplan, Jerome and Ford, Caroline S. "Rehabilitation for the Elderly: An Eleven-Year Assessment." *Gerontologist* 15:393–397, October, 1975.

Kastenbaum, R. The Reluctant Therapist." *Geriatrics.* 18:296–301, 1963.

Kosberg, J. and A. Harris. "Attitudes Toward Elderly Clients." *Health and Social Work.* 3:3:69–90, August 1978.

Kosberg, J., S. Cohen and A. Mendlovitz. "Comparison of Supervisors' Attitudes in a Home for the Aged." *Gerontologist.* 12:241–245, Autumn 1972.

McDonald M. "Reversal of Helplessness: Behavior Modification with the Elderly." *Perspectives in Long-Term Care.* 5:2 1974.

Palmore, E. "The Facts on Aging Quiz: A Review of Findings." *Gerontologist.* 20:669–672, 1980.

Pascale, Richard T. and Athos, Anthony B. *The Art of Japanese Management.* New York, Warner Books, 1972, 368 pages.

Reed, Julian and Gessner, John. "Rehabilitation in the Extended Care Facility." *Geriatric Soc.* 27(7):325–329, 1979.

Robb, Susanne. "Attitudes and Intentions of Baccalaureate Nursing Students Toward the Elderly." *Nursing Research.* 28:1:43–50, January–February 1979.

Rubenstein, L.Z. et al. "Effectiveness of a Geriatric Evaluation Unit." *New England Journal of Medicine.* 311:26:1664–1670, December 27, 1984.

Smith, Everette. Lecture. Exercise and the Aging Process. University of Minnesota, 1980.

Sperbeck, David. "Dependency in the Institutional Setting: A Behavioral Training Program for Geriatric Staff." *Gerontologist.* 21:3:268–275, June 1981.

Strayer, Michael. *Dentists' Stereotyped Knowledge of the Elderly in Relationship to Personal Problems in Patient Management.* unpublished Master's Thesis, University of Minnesota, 1985.

Wagner, Linda J. and Hilger, Sr. Brenda. "Geriatric Rehabilitation: Using an Interdisciplinary Approach." *Hospital Progress.* 40–42, March, 1981.

West, H. and W. Levy. "Knowledge of Aging in the Medical Profession." *Gerontology and Geriatrics Education.* 4:23–31, 1984.

Wolk, R. and R. Wolk. "Professional Workers' Attitudes Toward the Aged." *Journal of American Geriatrics Society.* 25:6242–639, 1977.

EXECUTIVE LEADERSHIP FOR ORGANIZATIONAL DEVELOPMENT

This section assumes that the administrator already has basic management knowledge and skills in hand. Texts on general administration, human resource management, organizational behavior, and financial management are readily available. It is more difficult to find information on the special applications of this knowledge in the field of long-term care.

For this reason, this section only deals with four aspects of administration, selected by the editors because they are critical to competent leadership in long-term care organizations. Chapter 4, Governance of the Long-Term Care Organization, discusses criteria for improved governance. Chapter 5, Executive Leadership, identifies the major roles of an executive for this field. Chapter 6, Developing the Management Team, provides a rationale and some guidelines for improving management skills at all levels of the organization. Chapter 7, Fiscal Leadership, provides a mechanism for leadership in participative budgeting, and Chapter 8, Managing the Effects of Institutional Living, addresses one of the most critical areas of long-term care administration.

Chapter 4

GOVERNANCE OF THE
LONG TERM CARE ORGANIZATION

RUTH STRYKER AND WILLIAM HENRY

INTRODUCTION TO GOVERNANCE

A Board of Governance, Board of Directors or Board of Trustees is a collection of volunteers who take on ethical, moral and legal responsibilities for an organization. The limitation on individual liability varies with state law. While an organization may carry insurance for the liability aspects of governance, there is no way to assure moral and ethical accountability unless everyone understands the basics of trusteeship and monitors its performance.

A Board should bring needed expertise, objectivity, and knowledge of the community to the affairs of an organization. Its members should be able to attract financial, human and public resources to help achieve an organization's objectives and provide a collective wisdom for its problems. As each member learns more about the organization, a well informed spokesperson returns to the community.

In practice, however, boards are all too frequently ineffective. There are many causes. First of all, there is often confusion over the relationship of a member's governance role and his or her own occupation, especially if the member is in some form of management. Many nursing home board members come as successful managers of a business, law firm, or school system. That success results from the development of good problem-solving skills. In fact, their problem solving skills have usually become habitual and almost intuitive. Unfortunately, these skills are applied to tasks that are inappropriately brought for board actions.

When these same successful people sit on a board, they find it difficult NOT to face management problems. They are called upon to face governance problems which, in contrast, are less clearly defined, have no clear right and wrong answers, have few criteria for judging success, and often involve far reaching long range outcomes.

Psychologists call this "negative transfer." If a subject learns to do Task A, that learning interferes with the subject's ability to perform Task B. Experienced World War II bomber pilots took longer to learn to fly fighter planes than did less experienced pilots because they had to "unlearn" a prior set of skills before they could learn the new set. In health care governance, we see examples of negative transfer whenever the successful manager sitting on a board tries to manage, rather than govern the organization.

A second source of difficulty is a misperception of what the long term care facility is and should be. At any one time, it must be viewed as a public, caregiving institution, usually charity-oriented, and a business enterprise. Each board member must learn to speak to all perspectives, not just the one he or she knows best.

Finally, a board must be clear about to whom it is accountable. Is it a special constituency? Is it the community? Is it the residents? How does what is best for the organization fit in with what is best for the community?

What then does a board do? The primary function of a board is to establish the direction of the organization. What should it be doing? What are its purpose and goals? Where should it go? Carver says "Boards are the weakest link in the organizational chain" (p ii). He says this because governors often get into management's business, not because they are trying to usurp that function but because they do not know what governance is and neither does the CEO.

A board must address the basic value system of the organization, provide vision for its future, enable proactivity, and concentrate on both the consumers and the ownership of the entity, always focusing on the purpose and direction for the future. In order to do this, the CEO must assist the board to understand its role as opposed to the management role. Indeed, this should be in every CEO's job description.

This means that a board must avoid spending time on trivia, short-term goals, reviewing what staff has done (as opposed to what they might be recommending for the future), and getting involved in petty personnel disputes. The "hows" are for management to decide.

The board must also monitor organizational outcomes. Does it achieve the goals and broad policies set by the board? Many experts in this field recommend that the CEO's performance be reviewed by the board. Usually an executive committee does this, and the evaluation interview is then conducted by the Chair of the board. Regardless of how formally this is done, the basis for it is the organizational performance. If the "hows" chosen by the CEO have accomplished the "whats" chosen by the board, then the CEO has done the job.

What about individual board member performance? The importance of board membership is gradually being recognized as a vital factor in the success of non-profit organizations. For this reason, performance criteria for board members need to be formulated. Conrad and Glenn suggest such things as 1) participation in fund raising, 2) number of board and committee meetings attended, 3) participation in ad hoc activities, 4) offices held, 5) recommending new board members, and 6) introduction of new ideas. In other words, sitting on a board is no longer an honor without obligations.

The ultimate responsibility for the effectiveness of the facility falls to the board members; if he or she is not concerned with effectiveness, no one will be. Certainly physicians, nurses and others who provide services in the nursing home are concerned with their own effectiveness, but that is on a patient-by-patient basis. The degree to which the whole organization is effective in meeting the long-term care needs of the community must be determined by the board.

The major standard against which that effectiveness must be judged, and the key statement of the right thing that the facility is pursuing, is the mission statement. The mission establishes the organization's direction and dictates its policies. Thus, it is one of the board's major responsibilities. Unless the board negotiates an explicit statement of what the organization is trying to achieve, it faces the risk of each board member holding his/her own implicit assumption about the organization's mission. Moreover, when the organization's mission has not been explicitly stated to the community, each member of the community will hold a unique implicit idea about what the organization should be doing. This absence of a consensus on the part of the board makes it impossible for the board to govern. Without a clear statement of mission, it is not possible to generate meaningful goals for the organization. Worse, the community will not know what to expect of the institution.

Given an adequate mission statement, the board must pursue their concern for effectiveness by asking a lot of "so what?" questions. When told that the organization provided 8,000 patient days of care last year, the board should ask: "So what? What good did it do? Is anyone any healthier or happier because of that?" Even when told that the home's cost per day did not rise from last year, the board must ask: "So what? Can we **afford** to provide care at that cost? Are we still achieving our mission? What is that increase in our efficiency doing to our effectiveness?" The board's task is to provide the most cost-effective care, not merely the most cost efficient. It is outcome (not just output) per dollar that must be their focus.

So how does the board decide on the right thing and how does it assess effectiveness? How does the board decide how well the home's output is achieving the goals they want it to achieve? How does the board measure the impact on the community? First, there must be an adequate mission statement against which to judge performance (a clear statement against which to judge performance), a clear statement of the **right thing** which is being pursued by the organization. Among other things, it should state what services are provided and why they are provided (how they relate to the needs of the community). An example of an excellent mission statement is shown in Table 4-I. Note that it provides a good deal of information about the institution but can be reproduced on one sheet of paper. Note also that it is devoid of jargon and can be understood by "the person on the street."

Second (and this should also be part of the mission statement), who is "the community?" Whom does the home intend to serve? Is that population the same for all services or should the board expect to draw folks from a larger area for some special services? Third, the board needs to know about the health needs of the aged in these communities. Are these populations especially at risk for particular illnesses? What services might prevent precipitous declines in function? How prevalent are the problems the facility treats or might treat? Fourth, the board must be aware of the other health care providers who are serving the same communities. That means they should **communicate** with them about what each facility is planning to do.

Fifth, the board has to have some feedback loops established with the communities they serve—some way for information on the impact of the organization's services to get back to the organization. These might include the following:

- Follow-up surveys with residents and families
- Formal and informal information from physicians **and** nurses, therapists, pharmacists, transportation staff, social service agencies, etc.

TABLE 4-I
WASHINGTON COUNTY GERIATRIC CARE CENTER
1988 Mission Statement

Location/Service Area – Washington County Geriatric Care Center is a community based nonprofit nursing home in _____. It primarily serves frail elderly residents of Washington and Lincoln counties.

Major Goal – It's primary focus is to provide a safe environment where self-esteem, physical and psychosocial function, independence and personal decision making are enhanced.

Services Provided – It is a long-term care organization of 75 skilled and 50 intermediate care beds, prepared to care for a broad range of chronic conditions of the elderly. Psychiatric, dental, podiatry, speech, hearing, and vision services are available by consultation and available to the elderly in the community.

Areas of Special Expertise – Because of its specialized in-house and consultant staff, the Center offers special services not frequently found in county nursing homes. It has been active in physical rehabilitation, assessment and treatment of mental disorders, and family counseling. The Center is developing special strengths in hospice care.

Referral Patterns – The Center normally refers residents with severe acute illnesses to hospitals. Those who improve are referred to appropriate housing and service agencies. Terminally ill residents are not moved to other facilities except by special request of the family and physician.

Institutional Relationships – Washington County Geriatric Center believes that sharing of resources and programs between health care providers is both appropriate and beneficial to the communities served as well as the individual organizations. The Center will aggressively seek to identify potential areas for shared service development in the community.

Education – The Center will support and cooperate in educational programs aimed at improving the health of the community elderly and the competence of its staff. It will attempt to maintain the proficiency of its staff above the level of other community nursing homes of its size.

Technology – While the Center will not normally "pioneer" the use of new knowledge, it will quickly appraise research and participate in research conducted by reliable sources whenever the well-being of residents is of major concern.

Religion – The Center is nondenominational in the provision of its services, but subscribes to the basic humanitarian and Christian beliefs in its operation and management. Catholic and Protestant services are available. It is open to anyone for care, regardless of race, creed or color.

Cost of Care – The cost of providing both general and appropriate specialized services will always be a primary consideration in evaluating present and future programs. Cost efficient services at a standard of quality consistent with or higher than that available in comparable facilities will be a major goal.

- Resident origin studies—where do your residents come from for each service? Why do they come to you? What do they expect?

- Voluntary health associations: heart association, lung association, cancer society, etc.
- Community surveys: public expectations about long-term care facilities in general, about your organization
- Health data sources: HSA, state department of health, licensing agencies
- Other providers: hospitals, clinics, referral agencies and institutions, sheltered workshops, society for the blind, speech and hearing societies, home health agencies and providers of housing
- Board members from diverse segments of the community
- Community involvement in board committees: long-range planning committee, facility design committee
- Advisory boards: for particular issues or where the governing board is severely delimited by law

Sixth, you have to avoid the confusion between image and effectiveness. A facility's image is **not** the same as its effectiveness. You can be very effective and still have a lousy image and, worse, you can be very ineffective and still create a great image. The home's image in the community can be manipulated by public relations, independent of effectiveness. Be sure you are looking at effectiveness and not image.

AN EXCELLENT SUMMARY OF TRUSTEE

Responsibility to institution and community is in a statement of the board's fiduciary responsibility by the Minnesota Supreme Court:

> In the eyes of the law, there is no such thing as a dummy or nominal board of directors. The law confines the business management of a corporation to its directors, and they are vested with a fiduciary responsibility to administer its affairs. As such, they are charged with the duty to act for the corporation according to their best judgment, and in so doing they cannot be controlled in the reasonable exercise and performance of such duty. Directors may not agree to exercise their official duties for the benefit of any individual or interest other than the corporation itself—(**Jacobson** v. **Barnes**, 176 Minn. 4, 222 N.W. 341), and an agreement by which individual directors, or the entire board, abdicate or bargain away in advance the judgment which the law contemplates they shall exercise over the affairs of the corporation is contrary to public policy and void. **Seitz** v. **Michel**, 148 Minn.80,181, N.W. 102, 12 A.L.R.1060. They may not agree to abstain from discharging their fiduciary duty to participate actively and fully in the manage-

ment of corporate affairs. The law does not permit the creation of a sterilized board of directors.

—Kay v. Homewood Hospital, 27 N.W. 2d 409, 411; 223 Minn. 440(1947)

GOVERNANCE OF LONG-TERM CARE ORGANIZATIONS

Governance of long-term care organizations varies greatly. Indeed, a typical form of governance cannot be identified, but it is possible to describe the more common forms of current practice and board composition. In addition, potential problems of each form will be identified so that administrators and boards can be prepared to recognize more specific needs. For the purpose of this chapter, boards will be classified in three ways; those that govern a single home, those that govern multiple homes, and those with special forms of governance.

Boards of Single Homes

Most commonly, when a board governs a single organization, it is owned by a single proprietor, a partnership, a church, a unit of government, or a fraternal organization. The board structure and interest of board members vary enormously.

City and County Governance

In some instances, city or county nursing home boards consist of all elected commissioners or supervisors. In this case, nursing home business is an agenda item, just as are schools, police, fire, etc. This arrangement has the obvious disadvantage of limiting the amount of time available to the affairs of the long-term care organization, and of course provides no guarantee of knowledge or interest in this area by elected officials. More commonly, county or city commissioners elect or appoint (from their own members) a special board for the long-term care facility, and in some instances, elected officials also appoint board members from the community.

Church and Other Nonprofit Boards

Nonprofit organizations sponsoring long-term organizations sometimes have problems obtaining committed board members also. If a board member's appointment is based on long-time membership in an organization or past contributions to the sponsor rather than the ability to fill an identifiable contribution or need on the board, the organization loses potential vitality. Administrators and board members must identify the knowledge and personal qualities needed for membership and attempt to have the sponsoring organization locate such individuals from their members.

Single Proprietor or Partnership Boards

Homes owned by a single proprietor or partnership are usually incorporated and boards are generally small with members consisting of owners and families. However, it is not uncommon for such boards to also include community members. Like other boards, the range of knowledge and expertise of members determines the degree of isolation or involvement in the community at large. If an owner board member is also the administrator, it of course clouds the differences between governance and administrator responsibilities and must be carefully considered by the individual holding the dual position.

Hospital-Based Nursing Home Boards

Hospital-based nursing homes may be part of a proprietary or non-profit system. They are usually governed by the same board as the hospital, frequently administered by the same board as the hospital and frequently administered by the same person. Many surveyors, accreditors, staff who work in hospital-based long-term care, and administrators report that board members seem more interested in the business of the hospital than the nursing home, even if the nursing home beds far outnumber the hospital beds. As a result, the nursing home may in effect be merely a hospital department. This is not necessarily due to board disinterest. If the hospital administrator places low priority on the long-term care unit or fails to address its needs, the board is likely to be less involved and less interested also. When both the board and the administrator view the long-term care unit as a separate entity with unique needs, it can then be free to fulfill its own mission.

Boards of Multiple Long-Term Care Organizations

Organizations that govern multiple long-term care facilities may be responsible for a small number of homes in a local area or many homes in a state or region, or nationwide. Many are proprietary, but some are church-related or sponsored by other nonprofit organizations.

Nearly all of these organizations have a corporate board, but there is frequently not a separate board for each home. In this event, individual facility and community needs may be poorly addressed because corporate issues are naturally the primary concern of the board. Administrators of such facilities need to work out a communication line that can deal with specific issues related to their individual concerns and needs.

Special Forms of Governance

State Nursing Home

State nursing homes have a complex structure of governance. In a very real sense, the state legislature and the governor can be considered their primary source of governance. In the reality of operation, however, a governor appointed commissioner, usually of the Department of Public Welfare or its counterpart, is typically the actual source of governance. Within the department, there may be a Bureau of Mental Health or Division of Residential Facilities. While department, division, and bureau names vary, the basic structure is similar in most states. As a result, the governing body of a state nursing home is mainly composed of directors of these and related departments that also oversee many other institutions such as state mental hospitals. It should be noted that such board members are also in a line management hierarchy in relation to the administrator. Decisions may be slower to achieve because of the intimate relationship with such a bureaucracy, but special consultants and many resources are more available for the same reason.

Governance of Veterans' Homes

There are forty-eight veterans' homes in thirty-four states. While these organizations are licensed by the state where they are located, their income is derived from the Office of Veterans' Affairs, state subsidy and residents. Administratively, they are usually operated by a department or division of Veterans' Affairs which may or may not be a part of a state department of institutions, health, welfare, or human services. Most veterans' homes have a board of governance, but some do not. When there is a board of governance, members are usually appointed by the governor from such organizations as the American Legion, Veterans of Foreign Wars, Disabled American Veterans, and Veterans of World War I and II. In a few states, the administrator is directly responsible to the

State Commissioner of Veterans' Affairs and has no other form of governance.

The Long-Term Care Administrator and Governance

The foregoing observations on current long-term care governance, along with a careful reading of the first section of this chapter should help administrators to analyze the strengths and weaknesses of their board structure, board membership, and board responsibilities. One might speculate that the entire entity of long-term care organizations could be advanced through wider community-member knowledge and input.

One of two problems are prominent in many long-term care organizations. First, the administrator may assume policy responsibilities by default if the board is inactive. This places the board in the untenable position of legal responsibility without actual participation in major decisions. Second, the board may usurp administrative responsibilities if the administrator is weak or the board is unaware of its real role. The latter erodes the influence and effectiveness of the administrator and tends to attract administrators who wish to function as middle managers.

Whether a board is formal and highly structured or informal and loosely structured is not necessarily an issue in terms of board effectiveness. Board effectiveness comes from informed interest which will provide direction of long-range planning, policy formulation, fiscal planning and enablement of creative programming.

Ward's 1982 study of administrator tenure (6.4 years—mean) in 367 Minnesota nursing homes provides information regarding governance that is rarely available. Among these homes, board members were as follows:

27%— self-appointed
31%— elected or appointed by owners, stockholders or their representatives
24%— elected or appointed by general membership of an association or congregation
 9%— public election
    3%—directly to the board
    6%—elected officials appointed to the board

Ward also found that there were no statistically significant differences between administrator tenure and bed size, financial performance, type of ownership or a board of publicly elected members. Of these, the lack of relationship to financial performance is quite surprising.

His statistically significant findings were as follows:

1. The older the administrator, the longer the tenure.
2. The higher the salary, the longer the tenure.
3. The higher the education, the shorter the tenure. (38% had less than a baccalaureate degree, 42% had a baccalaureate degree, and almost 20% had a graduate degree.)
4. Administrators of multifacility organizations had shorter tenure.

While these findings show that there is mobility of younger, better educated administrators and apparently fewer such opportunities for older, less educated administrators, it also suggests several areas of consideration for administrators, governing boards, and organizational decision-making.

What criteria for administrator performance should be selected? While short tenure is disruptive to an organization, what are the indicators of organizational stagnation caused by long tenure? How can multifacility organizations address the problem of short tenure of administrators? Why isn't financial performance related to tenure?

The latter question is addressed in Holst's study of forty administrators and their corporate representatives in California. In this study, administrators and corporate representatives agreed on the goals of a maximum census, a good cash flow and a minimum number of health department noncompliances. They did not agree, however, about administrator job performance or quality of communications between central headquarters and local managers. Administrators tended to rate their job performance higher than their employers and corporate representatives perceived communications as more adequate than did the administrators. It would seem that even when an administrator reports to corporate managers, more specific performance criteria for administrators and agreement on content and frequency of communications need to be developed and agreed upon.

Both of these studies suggest the need for communication between boards and administrators. If an organization wishes to fulfill its social and legal obligations for an individual home, the following questions will need to be addressed:

- Does the mission statement clearly specify clientele, services and organizational direction?
- Are board and administrator responsibilities clearly delineated so that administrator autonomy is possible?

- Do performance criteria exist for administrator performance?
- Does the administrator define issues so that board policy and long-range planning can be determined?
- Are board members selected on the basis of their interest, willingness to work, community influence, and areas of expertise that fit into organizational needs?
- Are lines of access and communication to the board clearly established. known, and adhered to?
- Are board members and the administrator agreed upon new directions and willing to risk more creative and forward looking programs and services?
- Are board members sensitive to conflict of interest issues when nominating new members?

Administrators, preferrably before accepting a position, must analyze what is important to them in board membership, structure, and responsibilities in order that they may function freely in their areas of accountability. If there are elements of a particular board that need changing, it should first be discussed openly with a trusted member. That member can then move to other board members and find out if they are aware of the problems and agree to alternative suggestions for change. This will take time, but if the issues are made clear, especially the legal and social issues, discussions and changes are likely to occur, but gradually. The administrator will find his or her job far more challenging and interesting when the board is actively interested in the areas that are truly board prerogatives.

SUMMARY

While the problems of governance are complex, certain criteria can be established. Board members need to be willing to accept their fiduciary responsibilities and concentrate their efforts on planning the right thing to do and evaluating organizational effectiveness. In addition, they must communicate their expectations in terms of administrator job performance and organizational mission. By the same token, administrators must accept their appropriate responsibilities, communicate knowledgeable "state of the art" as a planning base, and report on the efficiency of the organization.

REFERENCES

Conrad, William R. and William E. Glenn. *The Effective Governing Board of Directors*, Athens, OH, Swallow Press, revised edition, 1983.

Carver, John. *Governance*, Unit of study for Executive Program Long-Term Care Administration, University of Minnesota, 1986.

Hendrickson, Robert and Ronald Mangum. *Governing Board and Administrator Liability*, American Association of Higher Education, One DuPont Circle, Suite 780, Washington, DC 20036.

Holst, Arthur. "Contracting for Administrative Effectiveness in the Convalescent Hospital—Nursing Home Industry", *Journal of Long Term Care Administration*, X:2:35–49, Summer, 1982.

Ward, Wayne. *The Relationship of Organizational and Individual Characteristics to the Tenure of Free-Standing Long Term Care Facilities in Minnesota*, unpublished master's thesis, School of Public Health, University of Minnesota, 1982.

Chapter 5

EXECUTIVE LEADERSHIP

George Kenneth Gordon

The term "executive" has become increasingly popular over the last few decades. We are all aware of time-worn expressions such as executive wash room, executive suite, and executive dining room. More recently, the world of advertising has blossomed with terms such as executive home sites, executive automobiles, and executive car care. In these popular usages, it is apparent that the term executive has the connotations of prestige, high status, privilege, and special treatment. It associates the term executive with romantic imagery of an idyllic lifestyle.

This popular meaning of the term executive is unfortunate because the executive function in organizations is critically important to their effectiveness. Nevertheless, the popular meaning of the term executive is so pervasive and potent that it is very difficult to lay it aside. It tends to get in the way when we attempt to understand what the executive function in organizations is.

This problem is further compounded by the fact that the executive function is not well defined in the literature of formal organizations. If you check the indexes of standard management textbooks, for example, you will typically find that the only listing of the word executive is for a section on "executive compensation" but the word executive, itself, is not defined.

Despite the ambiguities in defining the word executive, however, a number of keen observers and researchers have focused their attention specifically on the top senior managers of organizations who usually, though not always, carry the title of chief executive officer (CEO). The publications that come out of these inquiries are mostly descriptive. They describe the activities, behaviors, and operating procedures through which the CEO carries out her or his role. One generalization that comes out of these studies is that it is hard to generalize about CEO's and how they perform their roles as executives. The CEO's include a wide array of personality types, demonstrate a diverse array of operating procedures, and differ substantially in choosing the organizational issues to which they devote their energies.

TRANSFORMATIVE LEADERSHIP

Nevertheless, there are some recurring themes in the literature on the executive which are worthy of careful consideration. One such theme has to do with the way the executive provides leadership for the organization. This stream of literature has been especially influenced by James MacGregor Burns who contends that leadership is the most widely studied and least understood of human phenomena.

Burns says that most of what we find in textbooks regarding leadership and leadership theory has to do with one particular kind of leadership which he calls transactional leadership. He identifies this kind of leadership in terms of the face-to-face interpersonal influence process between a leader and a follower or work group. Most of this kind of leadership is explained theoretically in terms of transactions or exchanges between leaders and followers.

Burns and his colleagues contend that this understanding of leadership has been developed on the basis of research conducted largely by psychologists studying the supervisory-subordinate relationships in formal organizations. The leadership theories derived from this research may indeed be very helpful for the new supervisor, but Burns contends that the executive does a minimum of direct supervision of people who perform the daily work of the organization. This in no way should be construed as a denigration of the importance of effective supervision. It is, quite simply, a recognition of differential task requirements at different levels in the management system. Nor does this exclude the supervisor from performing transformative leadership. It is a matter of priorities, balance, and the way various positions are defined in the management system.

Burns contends that there is another kind of leadership which he calls transformative leadership. It is this kind of leadership, he suggests, that people have in mind when they talk about our nation's need for leadership. It is the kind of leadership which we associate with names like Ghandi and Martin Luther King, or Churchill and Roosevelt. These are people who exercised tremendous leadership influence over millions of people quite apart from ever meeting them on a face-to-face basis.

In his analysis of this other kind of leadership, Burns says that one of the characteristics of transformative leaders is their capacity to listen to their followers and thereby to identify and understand their deep human needs, aspirations, and hopes for the future. These leaders are able to meld and transform what they learn into a clearly articulated vision of a preferred alternative future and a plan of action through which that vision may be realized. Thereby, such leaders draw people to that vision and the people enlist themselves and their energies toward helping to make the vision a reality. This also has the effect of transforming the follower into an enabled and empowered person with a focus for competency and accomplishment.

Burns says that it is this kind of leadership which we think of when we talk of the need for organizational leadership as compared with supervision. It is part of the function of the executive.

Burns also suggests that every organization, no matter how large or small, has a need for organizational leadership. It is a requirement of the family unit and the corner grocery just as well as it is of the **Fortune** 500 companies. Obviously there are differences among organizations in the magnitude of the requirement for leadership and the resources that must be devoted to providing leadership. But without the required leadership, the organization, no matter how large or small, is essentially adrift and its effectiveness is compromised. Executive leadership provides focus and direction.

RECURRING THEMES

The foregoing is a very brief attempt to state the core of the Burns formulation regarding transformative leadership. Since Burns published his classic treatment of the subject in 1978, the concept of transformative leadership has been elaborated in various ways and has become a major theme in the literature on executive leadership in organizations.

Futurizing

Another theme has to do with "futurizing" for the organization. This obviously has close affinity with Burns's concept of the transformative leader as envisionizing the preferred alternative future. But the futurizing function is worthy of more specific elaboration.

After his retirement as CEO of Blue Cross/Blue Shield, Walt McNerney once pointed out that the Blues were then initiating changes in benefits and new insurance programs which the company had started developing five years before McNerney retired as CEO. The point he was making is that in a company that size, the leadership has to be thinking and planning at least five years into the future in order to anticipate what will be needed, develop new products, communicate the upcoming changes throughout the organization, and negotiate the acceptability of changes and new programs with the array of stakeholders involved. He added that though five years lead time is indeed a long time in which there is a great risk that circumstances may change considerably, he thought that corporations such as Blue Cross/Blue Shield may soon require as much as ten-year futurizing in order to maintain their positions in their businesses.

Speaking of the same futurizing function and the potential for bad decisions, Peter Drucker has suggested that this is why corporate executives are paid so well. It is the futurity and the irreversibility of their decisions and the courage required to make such decisions that drives the executive compensation systems. Executive leadership requires courage.

Futurizing for the organization should not be thought of as an idling away of time. A former CEO of Sears Roebuck says that during his tenure as CEO, he **disciplined** himself to think about the organization for two hours every day. Out of ten years of that discipline, he claimed that he had made two critically important decisions regarding the future business of the company.

Goal Setting and Strategy Formation

Futurizing is also the key to setting goals and strategy for the organization which constitute another theme in the literature of executive leadership. The disciplined analysis of the future requires identification of and working through the multiple contingencies facing the organization as well as the identification of new opportunities. This is the discipline which provides the basis for goal setting and strategy formation.

The clarity of future goals and strategy for their achievement has a direct effect on day-by-day operations. Decisions are always made with respect to keeping the organization constantly positioned and repositioned for a variety of contingencies posed by changes in the operating environment while still maintaining the course toward achieving the desired alternative future for the organization. Thus, goal setting and strategy formation provide a framework to guide daily decision making.

Communication

Communication constitutes another theme in the executive leadership literature. The vision of the future of the organization, the goals and strategies, must be clearly articulated and communicated if they are to serve the purposes presented above. Executives see to it that this communication function is fulfilled. They refine their communication skills and become adept at persuasion, negotiation, and team building. There is some research support for the proposition that as organizations grow in size, the executive devotes more energies to developing the people side of the organization and communication skills become increasingly important.

Affirming Values

A part of the communication function is the affirmation and clarification of the value commitments and culture of the organization. This values affirmation function is another theme of the current literature of executive leadership. In this respect, there is a considerable amount of literature on how the executive imprints her or his own personality on the organization. Across time, the entire organization and each of its component parts increasingly reflect the value commitments and character of the executive.

For one thing, employees who do not agree with the values of the executive "select themselves out" of the organization. In addition, their replacements are likely to be people who fit more comfortably with the evolving value commitments of the organization. Therefore, as the personal philosophy, value commitments, and ethics of the executive are incorporated into the organization, there are changes in personnel, program policy, and operating procedures which leave their distinctive mark on the organization. One effect of this process is the consolidation of internal consensus regarding the nature of the organization and how the daily work of the organization is carried out.

External Relations

Another theme in the executive leadership literature has to do with the executive's attention to the external environment of the organization and the cultivation of external communication linkages. Obviously, this theme has distinct relations to several of the other themes, especially futurizing for the organization.

However, the development of external relationships embraces much more than support for the futurizing. One of the functions served is that of public relations. That is, keeping people in the larger environment accurately informed about the organization and its work. This serves the important function of cultivating constituencies and garnering their support for the organization and its reason for being. Without the support of external constituencies, the organization may become alienated and encounter antagonism and resistance with respect to issues such as access to resources and manpower recruitment.

With respect to these last mentioned issues, it is important to note that the external communication linkages must be established and cultivated long before a specific need arises. Walt McNerney and his comments on Blue Cross/Blue Shield illustrate the point very well. Every time the company initiates a change in policies or programs, that change must be negotiated with each of the state commissioners of insurance, the labor unions, the employers, and the health care providers. This constitutes an immense network of communication channels and that network must be developed and cultivated long before it is needed to initiate any one specific change. There is a certain investment of executive resources which is required to sustain the external communication linkages of every organization and that is part of the cost of effective organizational performance.

AN ALTERNATIVE POINT OF VIEW

There is a body of literature which says that the importance of executive leadership has been vastly over-estimated in most management literature. Salancik and Pfeffer, for example, did a detailed study of the consequences of changes in mayoral leadership in 30 American cities. They analyzed 18 years of annual budgets for each of these cities sorting out the budgetary effects attributable to the city itself, the budgetary year, and the mayor. Changes in budgets were taken as changes in amount and quality of services provided by the city.

They found that the mayor had far less effect on budgets than did the city itself. In terms of budgetary influence attributable to the mayors, the median value was 9.9% of the variance in actual dollar allocations; the median value attributable to the cities themselves was 79.2% of the variance. The researchers further note that the mayors' greatest influence (approximately 14% of the variance) was in funding for libraries, health services, and parks and recreation. The mayors' smallest influence (approximately 7%) was in funding for police, fire, and highways. Salancik and Pfeffer suggest that these last three budget categories represent essential services. They are areas in which there are well organized and politically active special interest groups. They are also areas in which historic and continuing long-term commitments place constraints on how much budgetary change can be made in any given year.

The Salancik and Pfeffer study suggests that the organization has a momentum of its own and that changes in leadership have a relatively small effect in terms of influencing that momentum. On the basis of studies such as this one, Salancik and Pfeffer have also been instrumental in developing what is known as the resource dependence theory. This theory holds that the organization's dependence on resources in the external environment and the relative availability of those resources are the dominant factors affecting organizational performance. In this theoretical framework, the leadership of the organization is a factor of relatively smaller consequence — in fact, contributing perhaps a 7% difference in essential aspects.

When youthful administrators are introduced to the Salancik and Pfeffer research, they are typically depressed by the findings. Why should they aspire to a career in long-term care administration when there is so little impact? What is to be gained by preparing themselves with graduate education and ongoing continuing education if it makes so little difference — perhaps no more than a 7% difference regardless of their level of education?

It may seem to some that it is bad educational strategy to introduce the Salancik and Pfeffer research with youthful long-term care administrators. Indeed, we have a strong tradition in the United States of emphasizing the positives. It seems unnecessarily self-defeating to introduce negatives which undermine the enthusiasm and optimism which are so important for the long term care field. Why project the politics of city government onto long term care?

However, the Salancik and Pfeffer research is of high quality and makes an important contribution to our understanding of the role of executive leadership in organizational performance. For one thing, the data presented in this research is sobering. It promotes humility with respect to the real world constraints on administrator influence as well as a sense of respect for the organization and how power is distributed both within the organization as well as in the external environment. A lack of appropriate humility and respect may lead to misguided expectations, frustration, a frittering away of organizational resources, and the risk of unnecessary disruption or worse.

Salancik and Pfeffer are also very clear in stating that an understanding of how much influence the executive can or should have and under what circumstances is absolutely necessary to a realistic perspective on organizational action. Without this critical component, the perspective is distorted.

Finally, the Salancik and Pfeffer research did not include any qualitative evaluation of the **effects** of the budgetary changes associated with changes in mayoral leadership. They simply noted that there were changes and their magnitudes. This raises the question of the effects of those changes. It raises the idea that the 7% difference is a vital difference and that the way an executive uses that 7% difference makes the difference between excellence and mediocrity. What if the squandering of the 7% difference in ill-conceived and misguided action is the hallmark of mediocrity while the mark of excellence lies in the stewardship and vision with which the 7% difference is applied. Moreover, let your imagination grapple with the impact and significance of that 7% difference when its effects are accumulated over several years. This makes the 7% difference worth striving for and effective use of the 7% difference is the contribution that competent executive leadership can make to the long term care organization.

CONCLUSION

Someone has said, "We were trained to be managers, but we are called upon to be leaders." This remarkable statement sums up in capsule form what it means to take on the top senior management role, the executive role, in any organization. It is especially germane to the long term care field as we face what promises to be an extended period of constricted resources and increasing competition for access to those resources. We may, indeed, be facing decline in terms of the constant dollar value of available resources. It has been suggested that in times of growth and prosperity, organizations can get along well with good managers. In times of scarce resources or decline, they need leaders. In this chapter, we have highlighted some of the themes in the literature of executive leadership. The intent has been to illuminate what is required to make the transition from good management to effective organizational leadership.

RECOMMENDED READINGS

Barnard, Chester. *The Functions of the Executive.* Cambridge, Mass., Harvard University Press, 1938.

Bennis, Warren G., and Burt Naus. *Leaders: The Strategy for Taking Charge.* Harper and Row, 1985.

Shortell, Stephen M., and Arnold D. Kaluzny. *Health Care Management: A Text in Organizational Theory and Behavior.* New York, John Wiley, 1983.

Burns, James MacGregor. *Leadership.* New York, Harper and Row, 1978.

Gardner, John W. "The Tasks of Leadership, Part One: Getting Things Moving," *Personnel.* November, 1986, pp. 20–27.

————, "The Tasks of Leadership, Part Two: Setting an Example," *Personnel.* November, 1986, pp. 41–46.

Pfeffer, Jeffrey, and G. R. Salancik. *The External Control of Organizations.* New York, Harper and Row, 1978.

Salancik, Gerald R. "Constraints on Administrator Discretion: The Limited Influence of Mayors on City Budgets," *Urban Affairs Quarterly.* Vol. 12, No. 4, pp. 475–498.

Tichy, Noel. *The Transformative Leader.* New York, John Wiley, 1987.

Chapter 6

DEVELOPING THE MANAGEMENT TEAM

RUTH STRYKER

INTRODUCTION

66 Administration: The Critical Long-Term Care Variable" is the title of an article written over ten years ago (Smith et al). Its message seems even truer today. The authors studied thirty-three nursing homes in Washington and concluded that the external pressures in the field of long-term care no longer allow a manager to be traditional, passive or merely reactive; administrators must learn to manipulate organizational variables in order to provide efficient and effective care.

Every facility is subject to internal pressures brought about by owners or boards, staff, residents and family expectations. In addition, every organization must respond to external forces such as the ever-changing political climate, new regulations, changing reimbursement mechanisms and community interests. As a result, the administrator is forced to spend more and more time dealing with the outside, political world. It is therefore necessary to leave the internal management of the nursing home in the hands of a qualified staff. The long-term care administrator must be competent in both internal and external affairs, but much internal management is accomplished through development of department heads and supervisory staff.

The success of supervisory (or department head) development is contingent first upon the administrator either having or seeking appropriate management knowledge and skill for himself. Personnel cannot function unless the administrator knows how to keep the house in order. However, the administrator cannot do it alone. He or she must have supervisors who know how to supervise. They are the connecting links between employees and management. They represent management to workers, and workers to management. Their organizational position makes it possible for them to block both management and employee goals without being conscious of doing so. On the other hand, this same position can increase the viability of the organization IF supervisors understand their role and are given appropriate training.

Likert's Linking Pin Theory helps us to understand the delicate problems encountered in having a department head or supervisor position which links management and workers. Envision 100 chain links (100 workers) in five groups of twenty links with each group attached to one link (five supervisors or department heads) which are in turn attached to one link (the administrator). This visualization makes the dual role of the supervisor very clear. He or she must be both boss (supervisor) **and** subordinate (worker). This somewhat tenuous position requires clear lines of authority, clear areas of responsibility and special training for the job. When an administrator places new employees in the hands of an ineffective and/or untrained supervisor, conflict and turnover might well be expected.

Management skill at any level does have two aspects, personality and knowledge. An inept, insensitive, devisive or untrustworthy person probably can never become an effective manager regardless of knowledge and skill. On the other hand, a person who is competent in a job, sensitive and trustworthy cannot become an effective manager without learning management skills.

In reality, when a person enters some level of management, that person virtually makes a career change. Knowing how to do a job does not qualify someone to manage others to do it. In fact, a supervisor may remain focused on the performance of the former job, because he or she does not know how to coach and supervise others to do it. A supervisor must become a doer of different things.

This position affects another area of employee-employer relationships: namely, union organizing. Frequently when a union initiates an effort to organize employees, the administrator is surprised. This usually results from a lack of knowledge about employee problems or a resistance to find satisfactory resolutions. Administrators must realize that such employee efforts (including strikes) are often caused by supervisors as much as they are by the organization itself. Grievances that never surface or go unresolved at the supervisory level deprive the administrator of crucial facts. If this is accompanied by poor personnel practices the stage is set for unrest and organizing in order for employees to accomplish what they could not accomplish without union assistance.

In other instances, especially in small organizations, supervisors are labelled "inept" when in reality, their authority is usurped by a higher level of management. On the other hand, a supervisor may be willing to take the authority of the position but be reluctant to accept the responsibilities and accountability of the position. Because problems vary by individual and by organization, administrative assessment is necessary.

There is also a ripple effect among departments. Each department influences the work, attitudes and inefficiency of many others. For instance, unreliable and low performing housekeeping personnel influence the work and work flow of nursing, dietary and activities. Poor food and erratic food service may influence food intake and behavior of residents which in turn affects their physical and psychological well-being which then makes nursing care more difficult. Poor nursing care influences resident behavior, which may affect attitudes toward food, activities etc. Understanding, cooperation, efficient systems, and trained personnel in all departments are interdependent. As one administrator said, "whenever I improve one department, it always helps other departments. The entire organization is better off, not just that department."

With these introductory remarks in mind, the importance of the supervisor seems almost indisputable in terms of impact on employees, the administrator and overall organizational success. This chapter will examine organizational structure, supervisory responsibilities and what must be learned to perform in these capacities. The terms, supervisor and department head, will be used interchangeably throughout.

ORGANIZING YOUR STAFF

Organizational Structure

Who are the key leaders in your staff? Each facility will have its own unique way of delineating leadership and responsibility, but almost without fail, it will be shown in an organizational chart.

The average nursing home will have an organizational chart that looks similar to the one in Figure 6-1. As a general rule, it shows the board of directors or corporation at the head of an organization, followed by an administrator who alone is responsible to that body. Then, responsible to the administrator, are the heads of all the different departments within the facility, all on a very long horizontal line depicting equal responsibility. Under the department head line may be figures delineating second and third line managers and other support staff.

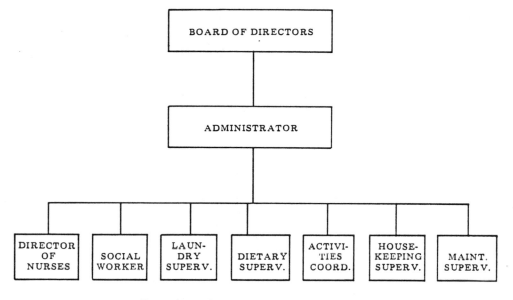

Figure 6-1. Traditional Organizational Chart

The number of boxes on the long horizontal line could be much greater, depending on the number of departments within an individual facility. The problem with this traditional organizational chart, of course, is that the various department heads or supervisors are responsible for unequal numbers of people. The director of nurses, for example, may be responsible for a department of sixty people, while the maintenance supervisor has responsibility for only two. This unbalanced delineation of responsibility may be a cause of conflict and certainly may lead to inefficiency with so many department heads reporting to the administrator.

An alternate organizational chart similar to Figure 6-2 may be better because it uses two lead assistants: a director of supportive services and a director of therapeutic services. Using this delineation, the personnel in the nursing, occupational and physical therapy, social service and activities departments would all be responsible to one person (who may or may not be the director of nurses). The remainder of the staff and their department heads would be responsible to the supportive services director. These two people would report directly to the administrator. The important thing is to arrive at a scheme that works well and then develop an organizational chart so that employees can easily see their niche in the system.

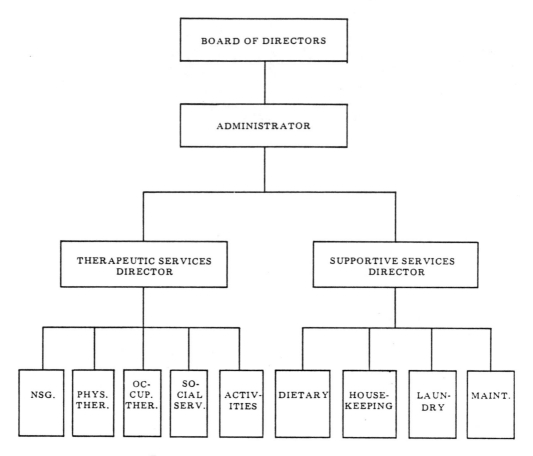

Figure 6-2. Alternative Organizational Chart

Responsibility

Once you have a chart to use as a visual aid, it is incumbent to make very clear to first level managers what responsibilities you are delegating to them and what expectations you have of them. It is unfair to expect members of a management team to perform efficiently unless they know what decisions and actions they can make on their own and which decisions you will reserve for yourself. It is also unfair to expect more of them than they are able to produce, so you should always keep in mind their educational level and experience.

Job Descriptions

Every administrator has worked with job descriptions until they are weary of the very term. However, they are an essential part of a well-managed facility. Here is an opportunity to sit down with a department head and very carefully discuss his/her responsibilities. Does the particular person have the opportunity to use his/her talents to the greatest extent? Has he/she been assigned responsibilities that are not appropriate? Do you expect your department heads to do their own purchasing and stay within a specified budget? Does the job description say so?

Job descriptions should include as complete a list of the employee's duties as possible. Not only will this help the employee to know what you expect, but it will provide a basis for job evaluations.

Delegation

We have spoken briefly about the importance of letting your first line managers know what responsibility you are giving them. It is equally important that you allow them to assume those responsibilities. Nothing is more discouraging to an employee than to be told he has responsibility for taking a certain action and to then have the administrator refuse to support a decision he makes. As an administrator, you take a risk when you delegate authority; but unless you allow your employees to make some decisions and subsequently support those decisions, your department heads will be of little help to you.

In the same manner, by delegating authority to your department heads, you are teaching them to delegate authority to their subordinates. When department heads see that they can successfully assume and carry out responsibility themselves, they are more likely to grant responsibility to their secondary managers.

Building up this spirit of trust and reliance can be very beneficial to the entire facility. When employees feel comfortable that they know what is expected of them and that their supervisors have confidence in them, they are willing to assume responsibility. Thus, decision making is not limited to the times the administrator is in the facility.

AN OVERVIEW OF MANAGEMENT LEVELS

Managers were not always managers. They have come up through the ranks of one or more organizations and held a variety of positions in those organizations. Success in previous jobs has culminated in their present managerial positions. The question, what caused them to be hired as a manager, must, of course, be asked. Was the manager a good cook, good accountant, good nurse, etc.? Did he or she show an ability to lead, to plan, to forecast, etc.?

Some managers will have been promoted for sound reasons: some for irrelevant reasons. Whatever reasons for advancement, a new manager, regardless of the level, must look at his or her new position in relation to previous responsibilities and those of others. One way to do this is to examine three levels of management in terms of job concentration, proximity of a manager to the environment where work is performed, the number of persons supervised, areas of planning and the kinds of problems for which one is responsible. See Table 6-I. One can see that a supervisor is physically close to the work situation in order to regularly assess worker and performance, job outputs and the work environment. This requires short-range planning and problem solving for impediments to quality of outputs or services.

On the other extreme, top level management is responsible for all parts of the organization, which by definition makes it impossible to be at multiple job sites and inappropriate because it would usurp supervisory responsibilities. This person's role with subordinate managers is more consultative, planning is long-range and problem areas relate to the future requiring conceptual and analytic skills. Examination of Table 6-I suggests the need for conscious changes and new learnings by persons moving into management for the first time and changing from one level to a new level.

From Worker to Supervisor

When an employee with expertise in a specific work area is promoted to a supervisory level position, the major change relates to a reorientation from doing to seeing that work is done. Learning can be obtained formally or informally, but requires the following:

1. Ability to withdraw from the doing of work except for teaching and role modeling purposes.
2. Ability to look for ways to improve efficiency, productivity, and effectiveness of all work done in an area.
3. Ability to coach and assist new and long-term employees.
4. Ability to rally a group of workers to cooperate with one another in order to maintain group identity and pride.
5. Ability to evaluate individuals on the basis of quality of job out-

TABLE 6-I
WAYS OF LOOKING AT MANAGEMENT LEVELS*

Areas of Consideration	Supervision	Middle Management	Top Level Management
Job concentration	Central to tasks, skills and performance of particular jobs and persons, usually in one specific location or a specific function.	Central to interdepartmental or multiple unit performance.	Central to overall organizational performance and future directions.
Proximity to environment where work is performed.	Close to place where work is performed.	Proximity unimportant because sources of information are mainly secondary.	Proximity unimportant as supervision of the job environment is delegated.
		May wish to enter a particular area where a chronic problem persists and other levels are incapable of dealing with it BUT ONLY TEMPORARILY	
Role with and number of persons supervised.	As many as can be observed regularly, usually daily.	Fewer persons. Role is to coordinate multiple areas/functions. Actual number relates to proportion of org. budget, proportion of org. employees, and number and complexity of tasks in each unit or department.	Fewer persons. Role emphasis is more consultative than supervisory.
Planning Range	Daily/weekly/monthly performance of tasks already determined by organization.	Monthly/yearly goals and subgoals to achieve direction of department(s)/unit(s) in relation to org. goals.	Joint planning with Trustees for directions in the next decade.
Range of problem areas	Solving of problems that impede top performance of tasks. Issues are predominantly concrete and shortrange.	Intermediate range problems. Anticipation of impact on personalities, new goals, etc. Flexibility and preparation of multiple solutions required. Issues are a mix of concrete and conceptual.	Long-range problems. Conceptual and futuristic with issues related to organizational role and function in community.

*Adapted from *The Managerial Woman.*

comes rather than personal characteristics unless the latter interfere with group performance and/or job outcomes.

From Supervisor to Middle Manager

When an employee assumes a middle manager position, the major change relates to a reorientation from technical (how to) in one work area to knowledge of work requirements and goals of two or more areas in the organization. Formal learning will be useful in (1) the behavioral sciences to understand peer, supervisor and subordinate relations, (2) the management process and (3) budgeting. The position requires the following:

1. Ability to work with the informal system.
2. Ability to delegate tasks, authority, and secondary responsibility to others.
3. Ability to conceptualize problems related to function of departments and overall organizational function.
4. Ability to assist supervisors to perform, analyze problems and seek solutions for improved performance at the unit/function level.

From Middle Management to Top-Level Management

When a person enters top-level management, the major change relates to a reorientation to overall organizational performance and the role of the organization to the external environment. Demonstrated success in moving human and other resources toward organizational goals signals an individual's ability to work well externally. Broad formal and informal education is helpful to the development of the organization. In addition to the requirements of middle management, this position requires:

1. Leadership skills
2. Negotiating skills
3. Knowledge of long-term fiscal management
4. Knowledge of new and upcoming public policy affecting the function and direction of the organization specifically and the field generally.

These conceptual distinctions between management levels should certainly not be viewed rigidly. Indeed, there may be fewer or more than three levels. However, the framework does provide a basis for analyzing the various levels of management in one's own organization. It identifies the needs of newly promoted persons and provides guidelines for a facility-wide management structure.

The supervisory level of management is likely to be fairly similar in all organizations and is crucial to consistent quality of day-to-day organizational performance. The middle management and top level management levels are frequently blurred in small organizations because there are so few management levels. This may result in ill-defined levels especially when the informal organization dominates. Larger organizations frequently mislabel the supervisory level as a middle management level. For example, if the middle management group includes a food service supervisor, the social worker (a single person department which is actually a service function, not a department) and the director of nursing (responsible for 60 to 70 percent of the organization's personnel, several levels of management within the department, and work performed in multiple sites), there may be many interdepartmental problems. In such an event, the administrator must reexamine the organization, not in terms of the importance of each (they are all important and interdependent) but in terms of management responsibility in the organization. If the administrator does not distinguish between management responsibility and a particular service or cluster of services, organizational success will be impeded by the structure itself.

Finally, multi-institution organizations have still a different problem. Institutional administrators usually function at a middle management level in terms of the organization and top management level of the institution. Multi-institution leaders need to think through these issues as they relate to delegation of authority, responsibility, and accountability at both the corporate and institutional levels.

One other potential problem needs to be examined by the administrator. If one level of management usurps or impedes the authority and responsibility of another level, organizational performance is diminished. This can occur at any level. For example, an administrator may usurp the supervisory or middle management level in a job once held. This diminishes performance of the person currently holding the position, creates mixed expectations for workers, and detracts from the performance of the job at hand. If a person cannot be assisted to develop new skills, that person needs to be replaced.

This can occur in reverse. A supervisor can impede the function of the middle manager by demeaning and/or resisting that person's goals and authority. Such situations may be caused by interpersonal problems or management incompetence at any level. In any case, this is why persons at all levels need to have a general understanding of the responsibilities of each level of management and specific knowledge of his/her level in particular.

PROMOTING A WORKER TO SUPERVISOR

According to Section 2(11) of the National Labor Relations Act, "The term 'supervisor' means any individual having authority in the interests of the employer to hire, transfer, suspend, lay off, recall, promote, discharge, assign, reward or discipline other employees, or responsibility to direct them or to adjust their grievances or effectively to recommend such action if in connection with the foregoing, the exercise of such authority is not of a merely routine or clerical nature, but requires the use of independent judgment."

In addition to the above, most supervisors need to participate in budgetary planning if they are to be truly accountable for their departments. The skills required for such a role are not learned in schools of nursing, physical therapy or other professional occupations, nor are they learned from being a cook, a housekeeper or a maintenance man.

While it is nice to receive a promotion, some people do not want to supervise others. Others may accept the promotion without realizing what the job entails. Therefore, it is crucial that job responsibilities be clearly described before a supervisor accepts such a position. While appropriate work experience and education about the work to be done may be necessary, willingness to expand into broader areas of responsibility is essential. Is the individual willing to accept responsibility for the work of others, to direct them, teach them and correct them? Is the person willing to participate in both budgetary planning and accountability? Does he or she wish to participate with a team of supervisors who help to establish organizational policies and procedures? Does the person have independent ideas for departmental changes?

If the person is willing to do these things, then the administrator must assess the individual's potential for the job and be willing to arrange for training in the areas where previous experience is lacking. Norman Metzger identified the primary range of responsibilities as:

1. Immediate leader of a designated segment of the work force.
2. Day-to-day decision maker.
3. Planner—short and long range.
4. Organizer of work, workers and work area.
5. Provider of conditions that allow maximum motivation of workers.
6. Counselor of employees.
7. Communicator—up and down.
8. Trainer.
9. Change agent.

The areas that trouble most new supervisors relate to interviewing, evaluating performance, discipline, use of authority and communicating appropriate information to staff. These concerns must be dealt with as soon as possible. When a worker is promoted from within the department where he or she has worked, there is a major disruption of social and group relations. Supervising friends and peers causes discomfort for all concerned. Especially in small communities, someone may have to supervise friends, neighbors and occasionally even relatives. How does one handle a good neighbor who is a poor worker? How does one become the boss of a former peer? Such problems must be discussed **before** a promotion. In addition, if there is any reluctance on the part of either the employee or employer (but they both wish to give it a try), the employee should be designated "acting" or "temporary" supervisor. Thus, if it does not go well, both parties will be spared embarrassment.

Time framed goals need to be set and arrangements for supervisory training should be made immediately. Whenever possible, it should be completed or at least started prior to assuming the position. Community colleges, vocational schools, trade associations and some large hospitals offer regular supervisory development programs. Administrators who have these skills often do it very well themselves. Readings can be suggested for independent learning, but there must be more to it than that. The administrator must be a good role model and coach the new supervisor, especially during the first few months. Regular conferences during the first few months will provide support and guidance when problems first arise with the new role. This also helps the new supervisor during the period when loss of the accustomed group identity is being replaced by a new more individual identity. In addition, it helps the individual to become acquainted with his or her new boss. Administrator assistance cannot be over-stressed. Good supervisors can help to protect the organization from a "them" vs. "us" posture between managers and workers, but both the administrator and the supervisor must work together to make this happen.

This chapter is not intended to be a supervisor's training text. Its purpose is to stimulate both administrators and supervisors to examine their own knowledge, to identify their own needs and to upgrade the skills that need strengthening. However, most knowledge and skill in most of the following areas will be required.

1. The importance of the supervisor
2. The supervisor's impact on an organization—employees, clients and finance

3. Interviewing skills for:
   Screening applicants
   Evaluating employees
   Disciplining employees
   Emotion-laden problems
4. The art of listening
5. Appraisals
   Objectives
   Work-related vs. trait- or person-related criteria
   Goal setting for weak performance areas
6. Discipline
   Legal aspects
   Disciplinary measures
   Effective methods
7. Handling grievances
   Getting the facts from all parties
   Writing up the facts
   Following the steps of the grievance procedure
   Staying objective even if you are involved
8. Do's and Don'ts of a Union Organizing Campaign
9. Communications
   Upward—employee problems, employee suggestions, unattended
      employee needs
   Downward—administrative changes (be ahead of the grapevine),
      organizational and personnel changes.
10. Basic problem-solving
11. Supervisory records
12. How to evaluate yourself

There are obvious other topics, but as supervisory development becomes an on-going part of an inservice program, participants will generate their own ideas. Because supervisors turn over, a basic training plan is required for new supervisors. A one-event program is just a beginning, not enough to maintain supervisory skills. Episodic teaching is no guarantee of applied learning. Regular and diverse inputs are required to improve and sustain skills. Follow-up and appraisal of these will reinforce supervisory staff to apply their knowledge to supervisory behaviors. When an organization demonstrates a continuing commitment to employee development, employees will find their jobs more stimulating and satisfying as performance expectations rise. The organization will be rewarded by improved efficiency and more effective client care provided by a more stable, competent, and satisfied work force.

SUMMARY

Department heads are the primary managers of the long-term care facility. They should be carefully selected, they should have a good understanding of their role as a part of the management team, and they should be given every opportunity for self-improvement.

A creative administrator can do a good deal of the guiding, teaching and coaching of the management team including use of materials and knowledge from his or her own continuing education, both formal and informal. Administrators need to know their department heads well, analyze their needs and capabilities thoughtfully and spend some time carefully planning their educational experience.

The benefits to be reaped from building a strong management team include increased efficiency, more confident leadership at all levels, and freedom for the administrator to pursue external and long-range obligations.

REFERENCES

Hennig, Margaret and Jardim, Anne. *The Managerial Woman,* Pocket Books, New York, New York, 1976.

Likert, Rensis. *New Patterns of Management,* New York, McGraw-Hill, 1961, p. 14.

Metzger, Norman, *The Health Care Supervisor's Handbook,* Germantown, MD, Aspen Systems, 1978.

Peter, Laurence and Hull, Raymond, *The Peter Principle,* New York, Bantam Books, 1969.

Smith, Howard L., "Administration: The Critical Long-Term Care Variable," *HCM Review,* Fall 1977, pp. 67–72.

Chapter 7

FISCAL LEADERSHIP

BARBARA PORTNOY BARRON

Who makes financial decisions? The answer to this question reveals more about a long-term care facility than any other single question. The answer reveals the philosophy of the organization, how the organization is structured, how authority is distributed, the degree of centralization or decentralization, and the management style that is actually practised, not just professed, by the organization.

The administrator in most long-term care facilities has primary responsibility for establishing a financial decision-making process. This responsibility may be in conjunction with a Board of Directors, or in the case of a multi-facility organization, with the assistance of corporate personnel. However, the administrator usually retains operational responsibility for the financial management of a facility. Some basic principles for an administrator to consider in designing and implementing a financial process and a model for a financial decision-making process will be discussed in this chapter.

What is meant by a financial decision-making process and why should a long-term care facility have such a process? There is nothing mysterious about a financial decision-making process. It is merely a method for an organization to utilize in making financial decisions and solving problems or addressing concerns of a financial nature. Why should a long-term care facility adopt a financial decision-making process? A facility needs a financial system for the same reasons that systems are required or desirable in other areas of management. First, it is more effective and efficient for a facility to have an organized method, a logical progression for thinking through financial decisions, analyzing financial problems, and handling financial activities or tasks. Second, a facility needs a financial system to insure that appropriate, relevant information is considered whether the administrator is making a financial decision in the midst of a crisis or in a situation with a more flexible timeline.

DESIGNING A FINANCIAL DECISION-MAKING PROCESS

An administrator needs to review and consider a number of principles in designing a financial decision-making process. This review should always take place within the framework of the administrator's own facility.

1. A financial decision-making system should be designed to facilitate the achievement of the mission and goals of the facility (in the existing reimbursement system). This means that a financial decision-making process is not an end in and of itself. A financial process is a plan expressed in dollars or numbers and is only useful if it is designed to insure that goals are accomplished.

2. A financial system should encourage wise allocation of dollars through a program approach to budgeting. This must include establishment and justification of priorities and expenditures. A program approach in budgeting means that the dollars allocated for the various programs or services should be separately identified. For example, the budget for a therapeutic recreation (activities) department should clearly distinguish between the expenditures necessary for arts and crafts, daily living skill exercises, community activities, etc., rather than combine the dollars for supplies for all programs and services in the same line item. The budget should also distinguish between the expenditures related to the maintenance of existing programs versus the costs associated with expansion of new programs and services.

   This approach to budgeting is important because it facilitates making financial decisions, including, if necessary, reducing expenditures, based on the degree a particular program or service meets department and/or organization goals. In addition, since resources are limited, it is critical that the budget process include the development of systems for determining usage rates and standards for supplies and equipment, and performance and productivity standards for staff providing services.

3. A financial decision-making process should promote financial decisions being made at the lowest level possible in the organization. As in other areas of management, the parties that are most familiar with the area or closest to the provision of a particular program or service are usually best equipped to provide financial input and/or make the financial decision for administration.

4. A financial process should be designed to facilitate monitoring, evaluation, and the implementation of corrective action on a timely basis. A facility's financial process is not complete after the budget is developed and approved or a reimbursement rate report is submitted. Too often, management staff at all levels in an organization will believe that their major financial responsibility is satisfied after the budgeting process is completed. A long-term care facility's financial situation is constantly changing and fluctuating. In order to insure that an organization is healthy and sound financially, the financial status must be continually monitored, assessed, and, if necessary, corrective action must be selected and instituted.

5. A financial process should recognize and be responsive to limitations and idiosyncracies that exist in most long-term care (Medicaid and Medicare) reimbursement systems. For example, in many states there are delays and problems with the length of the rate determination process. Therefore, long-term care providers often find themselves paying current expenses with the reimbursement rate from the previous year or an interim or temporary rate. Again, the system needs to address and respond to resulting problems such as cash flow difficulties.

6. A financial decision-making process needs to be designed so that the participants can clearly understand and define their own role, responsibilities, the financial time-line, and the relationship between financial activities and financial decisions. Participants in the financial process should receive education regarding how decisions made at one level in the organization, or by a particular party, impact on the entire financial picture; that financial decisions are not made, nor are financial activities undertaken, in a vacuum. For example, it is important that department heads understand the relationship between how staff is utilized, including staffing patterns and schedules, performance standards, methods of delegation, and the facility's budget and financial requirements.

7. There needs to be a clear distinction between the roles and responsibilities of administration, controllers or accountants, and financial advisors. The role of a controller, accountant, or financial advisor should be to provide financial guidance and information for management, not to make management decisions for the administrator. In many situations, accountants/controllers are allowed either directly or indirectly through financial recommendations

to establish priorities, actions, or decisions for administration. The contribution of a financial advisor is critical in the financial decision-making process; however, the process will be more successful and credible when there is a clear definition of roles. The administrator must neither delegate his or her leadership role to advisors nor allow them to usurp that role.

8. A financial process should assure that department heads, as the primary managers in a long-term care facility, assume a major role in financial decision making. This includes being held responsible and accountable for their role in meeting program, service and financial goals of the organization. In many long-term care facilities, department heads are held accountable for achieving program or service goals but similar expectations are not required when financial assignments are given. For example, the director of a social service department is likely to receive a goal of increasing family involvement in patient/resident care planning conferences. This is certainly an appropriate goal; however, the director should also receive goals regarding budget adherence and census maintenance.

9. A financial decision-making process should be designed so that general parameters are established in the operating budget arena, allowing department heads to retain the authority to reallocate or restructure expenditures within the guidelines. Assuming a department head is meeting organization and department standards and goals and is adhering to overall budget limitations for the department, the department head would retain considerable latitude in determining, appropriating, and adjusting expenditures. For example, if the original approved housekeeping supply budget contained $1,000 for plastic liners and $600 for light bulbs, the director of housekeeping would have authority to reverse the expenditures, i.e. spend $1,000 for bulbs and $600 for liners or spend the dollars for any items in the same or a similarly classified chart of account.

10. The financial decision-making process should be designed so that establishing service and program priorities for the organization as a whole within the existing reimbursement system is the joint responsibility of the department heads and the administrator. In other words, the problem(s) of reducing or adjusting budgets to meet reimbursement rates, limitations, or restrictions should be

a shared obligation, rather than the sole responsibility of the administrator.

ESTABLISHING A FINANCIAL
DECISION-MAKING PROCESS

Initially, the administrator must select the overall structure of the process. A basic structure, though the terminology may certainly vary, should identify the major financial components of the process, the specific activities and tasks which will be included in each component, the format or methodology which should be utilized, the responsible party, and time-line, including initiation and completion dates for each task or activity. A model for a financial decision-making process will be discussed.

First, the administrator should determine which components should be included in the system. There are five major components which summarize the type of financial decisions generally made in long-term care facilities: budget-operating expenditures; budget-revenue; rate setting; monitoring, evaluation, corrective action; and the purchasing component. Second, the administrator should determine the appropriate tasks for each financial component.

In the operating expenditure component, budgeting decisions regarding capital expenditures, salaries and wages, benefits, leases/rental agreements, insurance, utilities, interest expense, property taxes, supplies, equipment, purchased services, and raw food need to be made. Table 7-I shows a way to organize financial decisions for the budget-operating expenditures component.

In the revenue component, projections regarding the number and distribution of patient/resident days and the utilization of other revenue-producing services such as physical therapy or occupational therapy need to be generated. Table 7-II shows a method for making financial decisions in the budget-revenue component.

The rate setting component includes financial tasks such as preparation of the reimbursement rate determination report for the Medicaid Program (including a determination of a daily rate for Medical Assistance residents) and determination of a rate for private pay patients/residents. Table 7-III shows a format for making financial decisions in the rate (charge) setting component.

The component of monitoring, evaluation, and corrective action should encompass tasks such as projecting cash flow; monitoring expenditures, revenue, and census fluctuations, including comparing actual results to the budget; identifying deviations and unanticipated or unexpected financial events; evaluating the event or change and its effect on the financial picture; and determining and instituting corrective action when appropriate. Table 7-IV shows a system for making financial decisions in the monitoring, evaluation, and corrective action component.

The component of purchasing should include financial activities, such as determining appropriate product, service, contract standards; selecting vendors; and authorizing and processing purchases. Table 7-V shows a way to approach financial decisions in the purchasing component.

Next, the administrator must determine what is the appropriate format and/or methodology for each financial activity or task. Particularly in a financial process, it makes sense to develop standardized ways to submit, display, and evaluate financial information. This need for standardization becomes extremely apparent if an administrator visualizes interpreting and attempting to consolidate ten department budgets, each prepared and submitted in a different format. The administrator's task would be, at the very best, frustrating and more likely would become an administrative nightmare.

In developing a format and/or methodology for each financial activity, there are a number of items to consider. There is no "correct" answer for the long-term care industry. Selection of an appropriate format or methodology must fit the requirements of the administrator's facility and staff and the reimbursement structure. It is usually dictated by how the financial information will ultimately be utilized, both internally and externally, and the type of financial decisions which will be generated from the information. In other words, by looking at the desired outcome, the administrator should be able to determine format. The administrator will also want to consider who will be utilizing the information, both internally and externally, and the frequency of the utilization. For example, will the information be utilized in negotiations with financial institutions? Will the information be utilized in the rate determination process with the Medicaid (Medical Assistance) Agency? Will department heads use the information on a monthly basis for budget adherence purposes? Designing a format or methodology which is simple, clear, and easily understood and interpreted by the parties involved in the financial decision-making process is certainly a critical consideration. Finally, in making format or methodology decisions the administrator needs to determine the type of financial information to be generated by each

TABLE 7-I
FINANCIAL DECISION-MAKING PROCESS
Budget-Operating Expenditures
Fiscal Year-Calendar Year

TASKS	FORMAT/METHODOLOGY	COMPLETION DATE
A. Capital Expenditures/ Depreciation	A. Label and describe capital expenditures as mandatory, necessary or desirable. Propose alternative to purchase, e.g. repair and maintain, lease, rental.	A.　11/7
B. Salaries/Wages (1) Wage Schedules (2) Staffing Patterns, Full-Time Equivalents	B. Submit staffing pattern by job classification, shift, floor/station/assignment. Submit wage schedules designed on basis of performance and tenure. Provide research data regarding salaries/wages offered in community. Calculate full-time equivalents required for each position.	B.　11/1
C. Benefits	C. Forecast costs associated with maintenance of current benefit level (including premium or eligibility changes). Proposals for new benefits must include description of service and explanation of associated costs.	C.　10/15
D. Leases/Rental Agreements	D.–H. 　　Project maintenance of current status and costs associated with additions/changes, and submit documentation of rate changes.	D.　11/7
E. Insurance		E.　11/7
F. Utilities		F.　11/7
G. Interest		G.　11/7
H. Property Taxes		H.　11/7
I. Supplies and Equipment	I. Establish system for determining standards and usage of supplies and minor equipment.	I. 11/7
J. Purchased Services	J. Describe the scope and frequency of utilization of consultants and contract personnel.	J.　11/7
K. Raw Food	K. Determine the cost of raw food—distinguish between meals, nourishments and other nutritional supplements, and costs associated with special events.	K.　11/7

financial activity and how the information should be devised and developed. For example, in regard to specific financial activity, is year-to-date information relevant and/or significant?

The administrator is responsible for the delegation of financial deci-

TABLE 7-I(continued)
FINANCIAL DECISION-MAKING PROCESS
Budget-Operating Expenditures
Fiscal Year-Calendar Year

RESPONSIBLE PARTY(IES)

Department Heads:	As individuals, develop and propose budget for own department in all operating expenditure areas. As group, with administrative guidance, propose capital expenditures for facility.
Administrator:	Develop budget forms and methodology. Review and revise department budget proposals. Insure continuity between budgets and goals. Do research necessary for budget development. Develop general facility and administrative budget.
Accountant/Controller:	Calculate impact of budget proposals and financial alternatives.
Board:	Approve final budget and general financial strategies through adoption of resolutions.

TABLE 7-II
FINANCIAL DECISION-MAKING PROCESS
Budget-Revenue
Fiscal Year-Calendar Year

TASKS	FORMAT/METHODOLOGY	COMPLETION DATE
A. Projection—Number of Patient/Resident Days	A. Project admissions and discharges and profiles of new residents by reviewing/discussing historical information and outlining future trends. Project information on monthly basis for fiscal year.	A. 11/15
B. Projection—Utilization of Revenue Producing Services	B. Project utilization of services by reviewing/discussing historical information and outlining future trends. Project information on monthly basis.	B. 11/15

RESPONSIBLE PARTY(IES)

Department Heads:	Directors of Nursing Service and Social Service research and prepare census projections. Directors of revenue producing centers (such as physical therapists, occupational therapists) project utilization of services.
Accountant/Controller:	Project revenues.
Administrator:	Provide assistance. Review and approve final projections.

---

sions and activities by determining who is best equipped or prepared to handle the authority and responsibility. The administrator will need to determine what role, if any, the following parties will play: department

TABLE 7-III
FINANCIAL DECISION-MAKING PROCESS
Rate (Charge) Setting
Fiscal Year-Calendar Year

TASKS	FORMAT/METHODOLOGY	COMPLETION DATE	
A. (1) Determination of Medical Assistance Rate	A. Project current year-end costs and cost changes for new year. Predict allowable maximum reimbursement rates and increases for new year. Generate Medical Assistance reimbursement rate for new year.	A. (1)	12/1
(2) Medical Assistance Reimbursement Report Preparation		(2)	3/1
B. Determination of Private Pay Rate	B. Determine private pay rate based on budget projections, Medical Assistance rate determination, and market research.	B.	12/1

RESPONSIBLE PARTY(IES)

Administrator and Controller (or Financial Advisor): Prepare rate reimbursement report and determine Medical Assistance rate and private pay rates.

heads, other supervisory personnel, an accountant/controller, the board of directors, in the case of a multifacility organization the corporate staff, bookkeeping staff, line staff, and consultants. An administrator may want to consider expanding the roles and responsibilities of the participants over time in the financial process, if he/she is working with a staff with limited financial expertise, education, and experience. In other words, just as in instituting any major organization change, an administrator may need to gradually design and implement a financial decision-making process.

As the final segment of the financial decision-making process, the administrator must determine when financial decisions and activities should occur and be completed. There are a number of considerations, some imposed by external agencies and factors, others attributable to the operation of the administrator's particular facility. Probably the major factor in establishing or determining a time-line is the facility's fiscal year, as certain parameters are almost naturally established by the fiscal year. Certain time guidelines are dictated by such things as when staff of a facility are prepared to work and meet with outside auditors and the length of the audit process. If a facility's reimbursement rate report is prepared or reviewed by an outside financial advisor, the administrator

TABLE 7-IV
FINANCIAL DECISION-MAKING PROCESS
Monitoring, Evaluation, and Corrective Action
Fiscal Year-Calendar Year

TASKS	FORMAT/METHODOLOGY	COMPLETION DATE
A. Project Cash Flow	A. Develop monthly/annual cash flow projections. Identify areas of cash flow concern and establish solutions.	A. 12/31
B. Monitor Budget—Expenditures, Revenue, Census Fluctuations	B. Develop monthly monitoring system including review of invoices, payroll summaries, financial statements. Explain discrepancies between actual experience versus budget on monitoring summary sheet.	B. Monthly
C. Attain Budget Projections	C. Propose and initiate actions to correct discrepancies and attain budget projections.	C. Monthly

RESPONSIBLE PARTY(IES)

Administrator and Controller:	Prepare cash flow projections.
Department Heads:	Monitor department budgets and implement corrective action to assure adherence to budget.
Administrator:	Insure adherence in the general and administrative areas and to overall organization budget.

must consider the time required by the process and when the reimbursement rate determination report must be submitted. The administrator also needs to consider how and when private pay residents must be notified of changes in rates. The degree of experience and exposure to a financial decision-making process by key participants will certainly dictate the time-line that the administrator establishes. In fact, an administrator may wish to revise the time-line as the staff becomes more familiar and experienced with the financial decision-making process. Finally, the administrator will want to develop a time-line that allows the necessary time for the administrator to review and revise financial information and activities.

SUMMARY

The administrator must assume fiscal leadership for the organization. This requires clearly defined responsibilities for all persons who need to

TABLE 7-V
FINANCIAL DECISION-MAKING PROCESS
Purchasing
Fiscal Year-Calendar Year

TASKS	FORMAT/METHODOLOGY	COMPLETION DATE
A. Determine Product/ Service Standards	A. Design studies/tests of supplies and equipment to determine standards.	A. 11/7
B. Select Vendors	B. Establish an initial vendor selection system and a semiannual evaluation process. Include assessment of delivery process and schedules, technical abilities of salespersons, willingness of salespersons to provide assistance.	B. 11/7
C. Authorize Purchases	C. Establish a purchase requisition system including mechanisms for placing and processing orders, checking goods received against orders, approving invoices, authorizing preparation of payment.	

RESPONSIBLE PARTY(IES)

Department Heads:	Develop studies/tests for supplies and equipment used in own department. Complete evaluation forms during initial selection of vendors and semiannually thereafter.
Administrator:	Assist in designing and analyzing studies/tests and the results. Develop vendor selection and evaluation criteria. Design and implement a purchase requisition system.
Controller:	Assist Administrator in designing a purchase requisition system with emphasis on the internal bookkeeping process.

be involved in advising and decision making. Second, the decision-making process must be established with identifiable needs and goals, realistic time-lines, congruency with state and federal agencies, and a monitoring system.

Chapter 8

MANAGING THE EFFECTS OF INSTITUTIONAL LIVING

GEORGE KENNETH GORDON

What is it that nursing home administrators manage? And how are they different from, or like, other health care administrators?

One of the important differences from many other health care administrators is that nursing home administrators are, in fact, managers of communities in which people live. In a very real sense, they function as the heads of families or clans. Because they are the heads of communities in which people live, management is accountable and responsible for the activities of residents round-the-clock, twenty-four hours a day.

According to observers such as Erving Goffman, that twenty-four-hour-a-day responsibility and accountability has a tremendous impact in the way that nursing homes and similar institutions, i.e. prisons, residential boarding schools, mental hospitals, some convents and monastaries, concentration camps, ships at sea, military boot camps, function. Such facilities are a part of a class of social institutions which are known technically as "total institutions."

A hotel, for example, is not a total institution in that the management of a hotel in New Orleans is not responsible and accountable for what the hotel guests do on Canal Street during Mardi Gras. The employees of the hotel are not likely to be interviewed on national T.V. and asked how come they were not aware when one of the hotel's guests was being mugged on Rampart Street, or where they were when one of the hotel residents was making lewd overtures to passers-by on Bourbon Street; or how come they were not aware of it when one of the residents slipped out a back entrance at 1:00 AM dressed only in pajamas.

A hotel is not a total institution. The management is not responsible and accountable for the behavior of the guests. However, the management of a nursing home is in fact responsible and accountable for the activities of the residents twenty-four hours each day.

89

The fact of accountability is critically important. Obviously, it is not good for a nursing home resident dressed only in pajamas to walk away from a nursing home at 1:00 AM in subfreezing weather. No one will argue; it is bad for the health and well-being of the resident. However, a home that promotes rehabilitation and independence must ask itself: When are independence and accountability contradictory?

The words of a recent nursing home court case say, "Someone has to be held accountable," and they put that accountability on the administrator. Quite simply summed up, there is a dilemma in that to promote independence of the residents is to risk liability.

What is not immediately obvious is that there are risks both ways. That is, if you have a rehabilitation philosophy and insist on maintaining maximum self-determination by the resident, you invite maximum risk of liability, especially with respect to residents who are intermittently more and less capable in making decisions about their own behavior. On the other hand, you are taking incalculable risks if you are systematically conservative about minimizing your liability by minimizing the choices available to the residents. In this case, you are, in fact, choosing to reduce your own liability at the cost of inducing and promoting the resident's dependency on the organization and the premature (and unnecessary) deterioration of the resident.

The matter of choosing between the two alternative errors presents a constant source of ambivalence and contradiction among nursing home personnel. Neither error is acceptable.

For personnel who are committed to rehabilitation (in the sense of restoring optimum independence of function or of maintaining and enhancing functional ability even in the face of catastrophic disability), it is unacceptable to take a systematically conservative approach of limiting liability by limiting and controlling choices and opportunities for individual initiative on the part of residents. On the other hand, to allow rehabilitatively oriented personnel free rein to exercise choices with respect to the initiatives of individual residents is also unacceptable, especially if something goes wrong.

The nursing home administrator thus faces a legendary "catch 22" with respect to the issues of maintaining order, on the one hand, and promoting independence and rehabilitation, on the other hand.

Most nursing homes include in their statement of philosophy a commitment to maintaining and promoting the independence of the residents. Such statements are not only laudable, they are essential in a democratic society. Vague and long-suffering though our political processes may be, any institution which contradicts the expectation of optimum maintenance and realization of independent action on the part of citizens in pursuit of their own rights as citizens must be subject to suspicion, continuing criticism, and rejection.

The foregoing paragraph is not a matter of rhetoric or public relations jawboning. It gets to the very essence of the right of an institution such as a nursing home to exist in the midst of a democratic society.

The point is that when a nursing home systematically limits residents' choices and initiatives in order to control the nursing homes' liability, that nursing home has, in fact, diluted or undermined the rehabilitation potential in favor of maintaining order. It has lost its role as a health care center. Under these circumstances, employees of the organization are likely to sense that they are caught up in what has been called "organizational sin." When employees are forced to merge their identities with a job, to argue cases of whose merit they are unconvinced, to give priority to rituals they know to be charades, and act committed while harboring doubts, the employees are caught up in organizational sin. As likely as not, the outcome will be conscious or (which is worse) subconscious resentment for the organization. A nursing home staff in which such sentiments are abroad is likely to be plodding and mechanical at best in carrying out the tasks of the organization.

It is apparent that nursing homes and their personnel constantly walk a fine line between being overly protective of residents and thereby eroding their physical and psychological independence, on one hand, while on the other hand being open to charges of negligence if they do not take reasonable precautions to protect residents from undue risk of harm. Walking this fine line requires a multitude of decisions which must be made on a case-by-case basis. There is ample opportunity for confusion and misunderstanding among staff as well as residents and their families about how and why particular decisions are made. Misunderstandings may also produce among employees a misperception of being immersed in organizational sin.

In light of the foregoing, it is obvious that every nursing home needs to mount a continuous program of self-evaluation and clarification of its role and function. If we can clarify for ourselves what it is that we are doing and how well, we have a basis upon which to educate the general public and refine the social contract or mandate within which the nursing home must perform.

Over one hundred administrator/students have carried out such in-house programs during the last ten years at the University of Minnesota. While the programs were individually designed and conducted, they all include several common characteristics.

First, they were developmental projects carried on systematically over a span of no less than two years. As a matter of fact, in most instances the program has been incorporated as a permanent, ongoing commitment of the organization. Such commitment reflects the fact that what is at stake in such efforts is a deliberate decision to change the deep roots of the culture of the organization. This is an immense task requiring a long-term commitment, and this must be recognized at the outset.

A second characteristic of these programs is a focus on clarifying the nature of the nursing home clientele. As has been described in Chapter 1, the history of nursing homes, and most especially their evolution during the last two decades, is such that the general citizenry harbors profound misunderstandings, myths, and fantasies with respect to nursing homes. We should not be surprised that nursing home personnel bring the same misunderstandings to their employment.

Perhaps the most damaging and disruptive area of misunderstanding is the belief that nursing home residents are simply people for whom no one else wants to care, that they are unfortunates who have been abandoned by their families, or that the residents are living in the nursing home because they have nowhere else to go. It is critically important to clarify that the typical nursing home resident presents disabilities of such scope and magnitude as to be unable to live independently except at great risk; disabilities that have outstripped the capacity of family, friends, and public services to sustain safe, independent living.

Such clarification is not easily achieved because the historical sources of misunderstanding are so deeply rooted. However, clarification is aided vastly by communication of the emerging research on dementia and mental health issues in aging as reported in chapter 14. Similarly, there is invaluable information contained in the last fifteen years of research and demonstration projects on "alternatives to nursing home care." Perhaps the most important outcome of the research on "alternatives" is the growing realization that the nursing home population is more disabled and, therefore, distinctly different from the frail elderly who can be sustained in independent living through expanded provision of community services. There is a growing body of research indicating that there is little overlap between the nursing home population and other elderly people who can benefit from expanded community services, and that there is almost no overlap at the skilled care level. It is important in this respect to note a shift of terminology in the "alternatives" literature; some researchers now write about "alternatives to **unnecessary** nursing home care" or refer to a "continuum of care." These changes in terminology reflect the growing acceptance of the fact that as a person's disabilities mount and compound, it is likely that nursing home care becomes increasingly a necessity in order to provide proper care and quality of life.

Nursing home personnel have a right to explore such clarification of the nature of our nursing home residents. It makes a world of difference to them when they grasp the fact that nursing home residents constitute a very special population which prior generations rarely if ever encountered.

A third common component of these administrator-led programs is a sharply focussed and candid exploration of the nature of the nursing home as a total institution. A key issue is understanding the dynamics of organizational power in a nursing home and the consequences for the health, well-being, and quality of life for residents. Out of this exploration flows a clarification and realization that a nursing home is a power-laden organization with potent impact on the lives of the residents and that every employee is a conduit through which that power flows. Therefore, the uses of organizational power must be constantly scrutinized and the psychosocial costs of organizational power to the residents must be carefully evaluated and weighed against the benefits. Especially important is the realization that organizational power is absolutely necessary in providing a safe, protected, and supportive care environment for people with the kind of disabilities that nursing home residents present. The responsible use of power thus requires both humility and empathy.

The exploration of organizational power and the nature of total institutions also leads to the recognition that every aspect of organizational practices and procedures, daily routines, programs, policies, and activities has subtle potential for functioning as a two-edge sword. Unless all aspects are constantly monitored and adjusted appropriately, they are almost all capable of contributing to increased disability and dependency among the residents.

The focus of projects varies widely depending on the history of the particular organization, the development of key staff people, and the maturity of the administrator. Nevertheless, at least one example may be in order.

In this particular home, a task force was formed to examine organizational practices which were overly institutionalizing for the residents. The task force zeroed in on the fact that most residents were going to bed shortly after the evening meal and were staying in bed for 12–14 hours. The task force then set up a detailed study of when people went to bed for the night, when they fell asleep, how long they were asleep, and when they got up for the day. They also discovered that the evening staff had a well established schedule which determined when each resident went to bed for the night.

The task group consequently developed a program which encouraged the residents individually to choose the bedtimes they preferred. The observations on time in bed and sleep time were continued and showed that the amount of sleep time remained almost identical, but the amount of time in bed was greatly reduced. This, of course, altered the practices and routines of the evening shift personnel. It also uncovered the need for an evening activities program. In addition, there was a reduction in incontinent episodes, use of sedatives, and intercom calls for the nurse during the night shift. In short, one change in choices available to the residents produced a remarkable array of effects.

The planning and conduct of programs like this require a great deal of courage and some risk-taking on the part of the administrator. It requires, among other things, that the administrator be able to share his/her own perception of the issues and value commitments. The administrator must also be able to help and support personnel in a similar study of themselves.

Part of the risk for the administrator is that some staff find such a confrontation with reality to be unacceptable. It can be intimidating. Some personnel seem to prefer the historical myths and fantasies about nursing homes and their residents and do not allow them to be challenged. Occasionally, a key staff person has quit rather than come to grips with reality.

For most personnel who have participated in these programs, however, the results are extremely positive:

1. There is a great sense of relief. The personnel understand for the first time the persistent sense of conflict and doubt which many have experienced over working in a nursing home.
2. There is a sense of cleansing in that the ill-defined perception of being immersed in organizational sin is dispelled.

3. They develop greater detachment and objectivity in examining day-to-day practices, evaluating their appropriateness, and adjusting them for a better mesh with the needs and capabilities of the residents.
4. They are more attuned to recognizing organizational practices which have become unnecessarily routinized and perpetuated, especially practices which were initiated at some point in the past to deal with a specific, though temporary, circumstance.
5. The whole staff becomes responsible for limiting the accretion of ossified institutional practices.
6. They report that they are freed up to interact with the residents more spontaneously and support more spontaneous and responsive interaction from the residents.

All of these outcomes help to control the power dynamics of the nursing home and keep the organization's power properly tuned and focussed to accomplishment of the supportive, therapeutic goals of the organization. The environment which is thus created produces an internal control and an ameliorating influence on how the nursing home functions as a total institution and that is the basic purpose of the programs described above.

Some people find the systematic analysis of nursing homes as total institutions to be hateful and frightening. Others find an objective description of nursing home residents shocking. The alternatives to such analysis and understanding appear likely to be wishful thinking, confusion about our mission and function, and irresponsibility with respect to the potent institutionalizing capacities of the organizational power of the nursing home. The power must be responsibly managed and this should be a special area of competency for nursing home administrators.

RECOMMENDED READINGS

Anderson, Nancy. Effects of Institutionalization on Self-Esteem, *J Gerontol,* Vol. 22, 1967, pp. 313–317.

Bennett, Ruth and Eisdorfer, Carl. The Institutional Environment and Behavioral Change, *Long-Term Care: A Handbook for Researchers, Planners, and Providers,* edited by Sylvia Sherwood, New York: Spectrum Publications, 1975, pp. 391–453.

Bowker, Lee H. *Humanizing Institutions for the Aged.* Lexington, MA, Lexington Books, 1982.

Etzioni, Amitai. *Modern Organizations.* Englewood Cliffs, NJ, Prentice-Hall; 1964.

Frankl, Viktor E. *Man's Search for Meaning.* New York, Washington Square Press, 1959.

Goffman, Erving. *Asylums.* Garden City, NY, Anchor Books (Doubleday), 1959.

Marris, Peter. *Loss and Change.* New York, Pantheon Books (Random House), 1974.

Seligman, Martin E. P. *Helplessness.* San Francisco, W. H. Freeman, 1975.

Smith, Kristen F., and Bengston, Vern. Positive Consequences of Institutionalization: Solidarity Between Elderly Parents and Their Middle Aged Children, *Gerontologist,* Vol. 22, Number 5, 1979, pp. 438–477.

Sperbeck, David J. and Whitbourne, Susan Krauss. Dependency in the Institutional Setting: A Behavioral Training Program for Geriatric Staff, *Gerontologist,* Vol. 21, Number 3, 1981, pp. 268–275.

Tobin, Sheldon and Morton Lieberman. *Last Home for the Aged.* San Francisco, Jossey-Bass, 1976.

PART III

MONITORING HUMAN RESOURCE MANAGEMENT

Human Resource Management (HRM) is defined by Hall and Goodale (1) as the "process through which an optimal fit is achieved among the employee, job, organization, and environment so that employees reach their desired level of satisfaction and performance and the organization meets its goals." Human Resource Management deals with the ways an **organization** treats individuals. An organization is obviously a collection of individuals, but employees perceive vacation time, compensation, and training as **company** systems as opposed to an individual CEO's way of handling staff. At the personal level, employees also expect to be treated fairly and honestly by their immediate supervisor.

Human resource management is guided by the philosophy that there are methods of organizing and treating people at all levels so that they will give their best to the organization and achieve personal satisfaction while they are performing their work. HRM is an on-going responsibility of all levels of management. Immediate supervisors are responsible for performance appraisal, interpreting and implementing personnel policies, hiring, and orienting new employees, etc. Higher levels of management are responsible for compensation planning, record systems, hiring systems, and monitoring and evaluating all components of the overall HR system.

Frederick Schuster (2) studied the relationship between annual financial performance and certain HRM practices in 760 companies. He found a statistically significant relationship between superior financial performance and the following six innovative HRM practices; assessment-centered approach to personnel selection, flexible reward systems, productivity bonus plans, goal-oriented performance appraisal, alternative work schedules and organizational development. The use of HRM innovations reflected a qualitative difference in a company's attitudes toward its employees as opposed to the number of innovations.

Why then, do so few companies use available HRM technology? Is it inertia or complacency? According to John Donnelly (3), former president of Harmon International, it is because managers are afraid of losing authority. The typical organizational pyramid "not only limits the capacity for growth of the individual managers, but artificially reinforces the authority and the notion of unquestioned wisdom of the man at the top. We simply do not believe in that constraint."

Using Donnelly's approach, a good HRM program can be organized in a variety of ways. Because it is not economically feasible for small organizations to employ HRM management specialists, many administrators must personally attend to the HR function. In this case, an administrator might use a personnel consultant to assist in setting up personnel policies, developing job descriptions, preparing personnel record forms, setting wage and salary scales, suggesting appraisal systems or recommending other personnel programs. An alternative method is for several small organizations to employ a personnel manager. In this way, recruitment, selection and job appraisal methods, as well as personnel records, can be monitored by an expert at a proportionately lower cost. In other words, the human resource function may be managed by the administrator, by the administrator with the help of a consultant, by shared services, or by a full-time HR manager.

This section will emphasize the use of personnel turnover as a way of viewing the quality of HR functions and deal with other selected components of HRM, namely:

1. Personnel Turnover as an indicator of HRM effectiveness—what the research has to say.
2. Recruitment, screening, and selection of personnel.
3. Staff development
4. Personnel policies with special impact on employees.
5. Monitoring and evaluating HR practices.

1. Hall, Douglas T. and James G. Goodale. **Human Resource Management** Glenview, IL. Scott, Foresman, 1985.
2. Schuster, Frederick E. **Human Resource Management**. Reston, VA. Reston, 1985. P. 9.
3. Ibid, p. 23.

Chapter 9

EMPLOYEE TURNOVER AS AN INDICATOR OF HRM EFFECTIVENESS: WHAT THE RESEARCH SAYS

RUTH STRYKER

THE EFFECTS OF TURNOVER

Employee turnover has been studied in almost all types of organizations including hospitals and nursing homes. The insights from research and the many commonalities among organizations provide a great deal of practical help to long-term care administrators.

First of all, why reduce personnel turnover? What are the issues? Turnover usually has a negative influence on the effectiveness of an organization in three major respects: 1) financial cost, 2) lower quality of patient care, and 3) disrupted personnel relations.

FINANCIAL COST

Financial cost to the organization includes the time required for terminating, recruitment, selection, interviewing, checking references, placement, training and greater supervision time for the new employee. Overtime of other employees may be required during the learning period. Salary costs of new less productive workers and lowered productivity of the helping workers must also be added. While such costs vary with the position, employee turnover is responsible for five to seven percent of total wages (Boe). Of particular interest to nursing home administrators is a report by two hospitals that it costs more to replace nursing assistants than it does to replace either the LPN or RN because of the training needs and longer period of low productivity.

Health care is a labor intensive industry, accounting for 60 to 70 percent of its budget. Therefore, unnecessary labor costs cannot be treated lightly. While the replacement cost of different positions vary, the formula of four times the monthly salary is a useful estimate of the

99

cost of turnover of short-term employees, as suggested by the University of Southern California School of Business (Schwartz).

Every department head and administrator needs to think about costs. How many persons and how much time are required for paper and records that must be closed and opened for new and terminating employees? How much overtime is paid because of loss of one or more employees? What is the cost of using temporaries from employment pools? What is the loss of supervision time to employees when the supervisor spends hours interviewing job applicants? How much breakage and waste of supplies, linen, and equipment is caused by new employees? How much down time is required of other employees who assist new personnel? How many back injuries occur with newer employees? What is the cost of want ads, posters and bonuses for finding new employees? Every organization needs to flush out actual costs. Unnecessary acquisition, training and separation costs are unacceptable to a competent administrator.

Unfortunately, some administrators claim that turnover is cheaper because of the high number of base salaries and employee benefits. Research on the subject does not support this short-sighted view. Arthur Brief calls employee turnover "the greatest cause of fiscal loss in personnel management." The real costs result in failure of the organization to develop, the inability to attract good workers because of its poor reputation as an employer, and reduced work output and inefficiency resulting in low productivity during the never ending learning periods of new personnel.

REDUCED QUALITY OF CARE

Another effect of employee turnover relates to quality of care of residents. Kahne relates the acquisition of new personnel to an increased number of patient suicides in a mental hospital. Burling and Lentz reported a downward effect on nursing care standards when there was rapid turnover in hospitals. Revans reports a relationship between turnover of nurses, attrition of student nurses and length of stay for patients in British hospitals. Where turnover of nurses was high, he found that the attrition rate of student nurses was high and the length of stay for patients with acute conditions was at least one day longer.

The effect of high turnover on patient outcomes in nursing homes has not been studied. However, one must speculate about such influences on frail elderly residents who have suffered innumerable losses of close persons such as spouse, friends, siblings and children. It is entirely possible that depression might increase, the desire to disengage from others might increase, disorientation might increase and so might a sense of isolation, hopelessness and disappointment. Because personnel in long-term care institutions serve not only as caretakers but also as friends of residents, negative treatment outcomes are entirely possible. Certainly new employees are more likely to function at a custodial level than at a therapeutic level.

A vice president of a nursing home chain reports that quality of care is consistently higher in their low turnover homes. In addition, many administrators report a greater number of patient incidents with new employees. Concern for residents is an added incentive for administrators and department heads to become more attentive to a stable staff. While low turnover cannot guarantee quality of care, certainly high turnover makes it almost impossible.

DISRUPTED PERSONNEL RELATIONS

The third cost of high turnover is associated with the morale of personnel and their relationships with one another. Price reports that high turnover decreases staff integration. Work groups do not have time to form. The crucial socialization process of workers is disrupted by the constant coming and going of new members. Weakened agreement on standards of care causes dissention among staff and lack of uniformity of care. Loyal and dedicated staff who must routinely shift their time from residents (their reason for working) to assist constantly arriving new employees may also resign because of reduced work satisfaction. This is true whether the employee works in the kitchen, the laundry, housekeeping, nursing or activities.

"Stayers" may have a sense of being exploited by the extra load. In addition, morale deteriorates because of disrupted work routines, disrupted work schedules, and a sense of guilt that residents are receiving less than desirable quality of care.

On the other hand, very low turnover or none could result in a stagnant organization, devoid of fresh ideas and the stimulation of new personalities. Therefore, the goal of reducing turnover to near zero is unsound and probably impossible in any event. If one examines the "leavers" of an organization, turnover can sometimes have a positive influence on staff relationships and resident care. When low performers leave, morale of both personnel and residents is likely to rise. When the organization introduces innovative programming, new employee performance standards are expected. If employees block progress or are reluctant to change their performance level, they are not a loss to the organization when they leave.

Price reports that organizational development is adversely affected when an administrator stays either a very long time or a very short time. This undoubtedly has to do with lack of knowledge and inaccurate insights in the case of short tenure and the lack of vision and creativity as well as complacency that sometimes comes with very long periods of employment in one place. Thus, it seems that some turnover can be beneficial to an organization.

WORK SATISFACTION AND WORK PERFORMANCE

At present, research into the relationship between job satisfaction and performance is inconclusive. It has been postulated that a sense of accomplishment, recognition, belonging, esteem, security, personal growth and approval can serve as rewards and result in work satisfaction. However, Herzberg's review of twenty-six studies and Vroom's review of twenty studies concluded that the relationship between satisfaction and performance is a weak one.

Brayfield and Crockett suggest that high satisfaction and high productivity occur together when the latter is perceived as a path to goals that are achieved. Under other circumstances, they conclude that satisfaction and productivity might be unrelated or even negatively related. In other words, the relationship between job satisfaction and high performance does not seem to occur unless other factors are also in place.

Mobley and others consider job dissatisfaction to be "conceptually simplistic and empirically deficient bases for understanding the employee turnover process." Therefore, we need to know more about the relationship between turnover and job satisfaction. Bieter reviewed the literature in this area and concluded that the positive association between job dissatisfaction and turnover, as well as absenteeism, while "significant in industry, has not been adequately documented in health care." (p. 9). While her study was done in a large metropolitan hospital, it suggests several HRM behaviors.

The work satisfaction of 1435 employees was measured through a survey of ten work environment factors. She found only one statistically significant dimension, work facilitation. This factor was defined as the extent to which information, assistance, and guidance of a constructive nature is provided in the work environment. This includes the removal of behavioral barriers and obstacles to enable persons to complete their task.

Bieter's study fits very well with other studies. Price views satisfaction as a product of personal integration into the organization, a factor that would most certainly be influenced by Bieter's factor, work facilitation. It also confirms some of Revan's findings in Britain; namely, that turnover is related to the amount of anxiety experienced on the job. Anxiety in his study was reduced by many of the elements of work facilitation. Consideration of this factor cannot be overemphasized for administrative practice.

Compensation was not statistically significant in Bieter's study. This was also true in the Minnesota studies of nursing homes and contrasts with some studies of business. This does not mean that money is unimportant to health care workers, but it does seem to be a less potent factor when a person decides to leave.

While we can learn from business and industry, we must identify which factors that are particularly important to health care organizations. Arthur Brief suggests a model derived from his hospital experience and a literature review worthy of consideration by nursing homes.

He concludes that dissatisfaction with the work itself may be the underlying cause of turnover of nurses. He proposes that work dissatisfaction relates to the following:

1. Many hospitals design nursing jobs that do not provide an opportunity to (a) use a variety of skills, (b) perform all or a meaningful part of a task (too little identity with a task), (c) exercise discretion of work methods (autonomy) and (d) know the degree of effectiveness of performance (feedback).
2. Nursing education promotes the idea that its graduates can expect to find challenging and meaningful positions. When a nursing service department does not live up to these expectations, there is dissatisfaction and turnover occurs.
3. If money is highly valued and work is not satisfying, dissatisfaction may result in turnover.
4. If a nurse feels a responsibility to her family and work is not satisfying, the need to serve the family leads to turnover.

While the nursing home work environment differs from hospitals in many respects, these issues are not absent. Such a model identifies very specific elements that could be developed in the job itself to hold capable nurses and perhaps to attract a greater number of nurses to the field of geriatrics.

In another study, Seybolt and others developed a model to predict voluntary turnover of nurses in a Utah hospital. They gathered data from an attitude survey administered to 242 employed nurses (20% were LPN's and 80% were RN's). Turnover data was then collected one year later. Those who left did indeed differ from those who stayed. The leavers perceived little connection between performing well and obtaining valued outcomes which included opportunities (1) to make full use of abilities, (2) for autonomy, help and recognition from supervisors, (3) to learn new things and (4) to make independent decisions.

These two studies provide insights into the working needs of registered nurses in particular. Certainly nursing homes can provide these needs if the administrator is aware of them and willing to assure that the knowledge and abilities of professional nurses will not be underutilized.

Other useful insights come from looking at hospitals from the perspective of union organizing. The literature in this field was reviewed by Schwind. She found studies indicating that the institution's historic pattern of employee relations may be the single most important determinant for a group of employees to seek unionization. Equitable treatment of employees, opportunities to participate in decisions that affect them, a method for dealing with grievances, promotion and termination procedures, work assignments, shift scheduling, holidays, wage differentials (as distinct from wage levels) are considered key issues.

From this overview of employee withdrawal (turnover) from hospitals and other organizations, we will turn to nursing homes. It will then be possible to select more appropriate personnel practices.

WHAT DO WE KNOW ABOUT NURSING HOMES?

The literature on nursing home turnover is indeed meager compared to that on business and hospitals. As a result, many important and expensive decisions are made by administrators and policy makers on the basis of opinions and assumptions rather than facts. In any event, the lack of information on nursing home turnover stimulated two major studies in Minnesota. Available literature describes many problems, but there is a need to take information one step further—to analyze it for translation into remedial actions. That is what the Minnesota studies tried to do.

The turnover rate for all U.S. nursing home personnel was 60 percent in 1970 (U.S. Senate Sub-committee on Long Term Care). The mean turnover rate was 55 percent for Minnesota nursing homes and 26 percent for Minnesota Hospitals (Petersen). Nursing home turnover rates have been variously reported from 75 to 400 percent in California (Schwartz). In Utah, the average turnover rate of urban nursing homes was 110 percent and 78 percent for rural homes in 1970 (Kasteler). According to more recent studies, nursing homes have not changed in the 1980's.

Nursing home residents still receive about 80 to 90 percent of their care from nursing assistants rather than professional staff. A study of nursing home administrators in Pennsylvania indicated that "obtaining and/or keeping qualified help" was their most important problem (Pecarchik and Nelson). Fifty percent of the complaints against nursing homes in the state of Texas are caused by unlicensed, uncontrolled, health care workers.

A consultant for a chain of twenty-six nursing homes interviewed 400 past and present employees to determine the causes of turnover. The reasons for leaving were given in the following order of importance: 1) insufficient orientation, 2) difficulty on the job, 3) limited career ladder opportunities. 4) insufficient recognition of work well done, 5) inability to do the job and insufficient inservice education, 6) money, although the most unskilled indicated they were paid exactly what they were worth, and 7) difficulty with supervisors who were untrained in personnel management (Bales).

Training, and especially supervision, are dealt with infrequently. Pecarchik and Mather conclude the inservice personnel in nursing homes are often unqualified as educators. Staff turnover on a geriatric unit of a state mental hospital dropped from 76 to 49 percent during the first six months after an eighteen-session training program on the ward (Hickey). Inadequate supervision was described or implied in several studies (Molberg, Schwartz, Pecarchik, and Nelson). This seems almost predictable when one considers the minimal number of licensed nursing personnel required for intermediate and skilled facilities.

Current nursing home studies raise many questions. For instance, what caused the turnover variance found by Schwartz (75% to 400% in California) and Petersen (0% to 728% in Minnesota)? What was different about the homes on each end of the spectra? Why does one study suggest that fringe benefits and health care benefits cause problems while another concludes that weekends off, choice of shift and differential pay for weekend work is important?

It seems fairly evident that turnover resulted from one set of circumstances in one home and from a different set of circumstances in another home. Certainly, if the pay scale is low, that will encourage low level workers to come and go. If the pay scale is reasonably adequate, then fringe benefits become important. These studies lead us to a basic premise; namely, turnover is caused by a combination of factors which vary from one institution to another, but nearly all can be corrected by the administrator.

THE 1977 MINNESOTA STUDY

In 1977, 35 percent of Minnesota's 443 nursing homes were randomly selected for study of turnover on the basis of size, location and ownership. Over 30 variables were tested for association with the total facility turnover (FTO) and nursing assistant turnover rate only (NATO) using the Chi square test of statistical significance.

As expected, most homes had higher turnover for nursing assistants than for the total facility. Turnover rates varied greatly, ranging from 3 percent to 156 percent for N.A.T.O. and from 2 to 127 percent for F.T.O. Overall, the majority of homes had lower turnover rates than expected.

Both F.T.O. and N.A.T.O. were higher in larger communities, in proprietary homes, in larger homes and in homes with no life safety code orders. F.T.O. was lower when there were fewer SNF beds and in homes **without** JCAH accreditation.

Salary, number of ICF or SNF beds, number of license orders, presence of unions, and number of orientation days were not statistically significant at the .05 level of confidence, nor were any administrator variables.

The variables that are not significantly associated with turnover in this study were provocative. They may at least serve as deterrents to quick external interventions that may have little or no impact on the problem. Indeed, efforts directed at the internal factors of high turnover are likely to be far more effective.

The data from this survey suggest the following administrator interventions:

1. Maintain monthly records of characteristics of leavers and stayers, reasons for leaving, and turnover in each facility.

2. Strengthen the selection process of new employees by analysis of facility findings.
3. Examine turnover data whenever there is a change in salary, rotation of work schedule, change of work unit, change in part-time to full-time ratios, length of training, etc., to assess the effect on turnover.
4. Report part-time high school students separately from other part-time employees.
5. Examine the dynamics of the environment where employees tend to stay and leave.

Keith Petersen replicated the above study using 151 hospitals and 247 nursing homes, representing 86 percent of the hospitals and 69 percent of the nursing homes in Minnesota. The difference between hospital and nursing home turnover was again demonstrated. The range of turnover for hospitals was 2%–76% (FTO) and 0%–400% (NATO). The range of turnover for nursing homes was 0%–240% (FTO) and 0%–728% (NATO).

ADMINISTRATOR INTERVENTION STUDY

Previous studies described what existed. Next, it was time to see what could be done by administrators to reduce turnover. Emphasizing unavoidable factors such as size or location leads administrators to believe they are helpless or to excuse high turnover. This is untenable. Too many questions go begging. Why do some homes in large communities have low turnover? Why do some proprietary homes have low turnover? Why do some large homes have low turnover? To answer these questions, it seemed logical to study high turnover homes. The goal was to determine which administrative interventions would be most successful in reducing turnover.

Among 80 nursing homes within a 75-mile radius of the Twin City Metropolitan area, 37 met the one criterion for participation in this study; namely, a turnover rate of 70 percent or higher. The study lasted for two years, and each home was required to 1) send a representative to two seminars on turnover, 2) monitor its turnover quarterly for two years, 3) submit quarterly turnover reports to the author and 4) implement at least six administrative interventions during the two years.

Thirty-two of the 37 homes agreed to enter the study, but only 19 remained in the study for the full two years. Of these, 9 were non-profit and 10 were proprietary. The reasons given by the 13 homes that dropped out were "too much work" (3), "too many internal problems" (2), "change of administrator" (2), "there's nothing you can do about turnover" (2), and four gave no reason.

Two of the above homes are worth special note as they remained in the study for 18 of the 24 months. In one instance, the administrator had managed to reduce the turnover rate from 113 percent to 46 percent by the end of the first year. When the home was sold, the administrator resigned and the new administrator felt the problem had been solved.

In the second instance, the administrator worked very hard to reduce the turnover rate from 87 percent to 66 percent by the end of 15 months. The turnover jumped to 45 percent (180% annual if this had persisted) the following quarter. When I asked him what caused the sudden increase, he stated that the owner walked in one day and fired the director of nurses. Many personnel resigned in protest, as did the administrator.

Table 9-1 presents the prestudy turnover rate, the rate at the end of the second year of the study, the amount of change and the percent of change for all homes. The percent of change was calculated in order to relate the amount of change to the beginning turnover rate. For example, compare home number 6 with number 9. They ended with virtually the same turnover rate (60 vs. 63 percent). However, home 9 reduced its turnover by 40 percent while home 6 only reduced its turnover 10 percent.

For the final analysis, the top 7 homes with a change of 39 percent or higher were classified as successful homes and the last 7 homes with a change of 10 percent or less were classified as unsuccessful homes. It should be noted that the last 3 homes increased their turnover rates.

The 5 moderately successful homes considered themselves successful also. Indeed, they were better off. All of them reduced their turnover, in some instances quite substantially (see home 7 ending with a 59 percent turnover rate) and all but one ended with a turnover rate of 66 percent or less which would have prohibited their participation in the study initially. However, they were not classified as successful because the change was not great enough for statistical purposes of the study.

Five administrative interventions distinguished the successful from the unsuccessful homes at a significant statistical level. They were (1) increased supervision of new employees, (2) revised personnel policies, (3) increased recruiting measures, (4) supervisory training and (5) avoidance of use of personnel pools (homes in outlying areas unserved by pools were excluded for this calculation). Table 9-2 shows the differences between the interventions of the successful and unsuccessful homes.

Table 9-1
CHANGE IN TURNOVER—
PRESTUDY RATE COMPARED TO RATE
DURING SECOND YEAR OF STUDY

Classification	Home No.	Owner	Prestudy Turnover	Turnover 2nd Study Year	Amount Of Change	% of Change
7 homes	1	P	217%	53%	−164	−76%
classified	9	NP	100%	60%	− 40	−40%
successful	11	P	78%	39%	− 39	−50%
	8	NP	81%	45%	− 36	−44%
	10	P	83%	50%	− 33	−40%
	5	NP	81%	49%	− 32	−40%
	3	NP	70%	43%	− 27	−39%
5 homes	12	P	88%	64%	− 24	−27%
moderately	4	NP	84%	61%	− 23	−27%
successful	7	NP	79%	59%	− 20	−25%
	2	NP	81%	66%	− 15	−19%
	15	P	92%	80%	− 12	−14%
7 homes	6	P	70%	63%	− 7	−10%
classified	13	NP	77%	70%	− 7	− 9%
unsuccessful	17	P	84%	79%	− 5	− 6%
	19	P	85%	80%	− 5	− 6%
	16	P	80%	81%	+ 1	+ 1%
	18	P	73%	85%	+ 12	+16%
	14	NP	77%	94%	+ 17	+22%

This Table clearly shows several major differences in the two groups. First of all, successful homes mounted more effort as evidenced by the greater number and greater variety of interventions (71 vs. 34 interventions or 10.1 per home vs. 4.8 per home). For the significant variables, there is even a more striking difference, 35 interventions by the 7 successful homes compared to 9 of the same interventions by the 7 unsuccessful homes (4.7 per home vs. 1.2 per home).

This seems to confirm the need for multiple administrative actions because of the interrelated effects of these actions. In addition, it suggests a priority for certain ones. If high turnover begets high turnover, the same can be said for low turnover; low turnover promotes low turnover. The goal is to break into the cycle in as many ways as possible. If just 1 or 2 interventions worked, why was the home that both avoided the use of personnel pools and provided supervisory training unsuccessful? A brief examination of the relationship between one of the significant variables and the other four may help to explain this phenomenon.

Creative Long-Term Care Administration

Table 9-2

COMPARISON OF ADMINISTRATIVE INTERVENTIONS OF
SEVEN SUCCESSFUL AND SEVEN UNSUCCESSFUL NURSING HOMES

INTERVENTIONS	SUCCESSFUL							UNSUCCESSFUL						
	7	6	5	4	3	2	1	1	2	3	4	5	6	7
Revised Personnel Policies*														
Increased Recruitment*														
Supervisor Training*														
Avoidance of Pools†														
Increased Supervision*														
Exit Interviews														
Increased Orientation														
Primary Nursing														
Increased Staff														
Increased Inservice														
Employee Recognition														
Hired Personnel Director														
Employee Committee														
Master Staffing/sched. change														
Enforced Rules														
Replaced NA with LPN														
Bonus System														

	SUCCESSFUL	UNSUCCESSFUL
Significant Interventions	33 (4.7/home)	9 (1.2/home)
Other Interventions	38 (5.4/home)	25 (3.6/home)
Total Interventions	71 (10.1/home)	34 (4.8/home)

*Fisher exact significant at the .025 level

† Fisher exact significant at the .05 level for all metropolitan and suburban homes

Training of supervisors and department heads apparently will not reduce turnover unless the content is appropriate and other factors are in place. New employees require a significant amount of supervision. A supervisor training program may not help unless it includes techniques for supporting employees.

The frequent use of pool personnel constantly introduces new employees who do not know the work routines, the residents or the standards of the organization, and the supervisor has little or no authority over a person employed by another organization. In addition, it disrupts the group relations of regular employees and produces many of the same problems that a new employee does. Hoped for outcomes of supervisory training can also be hampered when inappropriate personnel are hired. The latter comes about when recruitment efforts do not provide enough available applicants to permit choices for employee selection. Finally, supervisory training cannot compensate for lack of direction when personnel policies are unclear, unwritten or unfair.

There are also interactions between the statistically significant variables and the other variables. Certainly little orientation, ineffective inservice and unpredictable work schedules can counter or diminish the effect of other interventions.

At this juncture, one might speculate about the unsuccessful homes. Did they consider the significant variables unimportant? Did they believe that high turnover could be reduced easily? Or did they believe that most turnover was inevitable and therefore do less? Whatever the reason, 3 of the unsuccessful homes did none of the significant interventions, 1 did one, 1 did 2 and 2 did 3. In contrast, 5 successful homes did all 5 significant interventions and 2 did 4 of the 5.

It is important to underscore that this study examined internal organizational factors that could be rectified by administrative action. Many other studies examined factors that are impossible or very difficult to change.

DEPARTMENTAL DIFFERENCES

The nursing department should be examined in terms of numbers and proportional contribution to the organization's turnover. If 70 percent of the total staff is in the nursing department, but it only contributes to 50 percent of the organization's turnover, then other departments (30 percent of the total staff) are contributing 50 percent also. In 8 of the 18 homes, nursing departments were not the major contributors to the problem. In order of frequency, the dietary department reported the highest turnover most frequently, the housekeeping department the second most frequently and nursing was the third most frequently reported.

WHEN AND WHY THEY LEFT

The 4,482 persons who left the 19 organizations during the two-year study period, left for the following reasons:

> 24% — personal reasons
> 28% — job competition
> 11% — returned to school
> 17% — job caused
> 20% — discharged or did not show up

While the reason for leaving and the reason given for leaving may not always be the same, it at least is information that administrators can study. For instance, if only 16 percent leave for personal reasons, this may be a part of unavoidable turnover, but if 41 percent leave for personal reasons, one might question if the screening interview was done well or if the real reason was not obtained. If 19 percent leave because of job competition, it may be caused by upward mobility and better salary and benefits elsewhere; but if 40 percent leave for this reason, one may need to examine the organization's hour, wage and benefit schedules, personnel policies, etc. The number of persons who return to school of course indicates the number of school-age employees who are hired. In order to regulate this, one might wish to place a ceiling on the number of positions to be filled by this part of the labor pool.

Job-caused terminations and discharges are more obviously related to organizational problems. Both reasons particularly relate to the screening interview, realistic statements of job expectations, salaries, quality of induction to the organization and supervision on the job.

Most leavers terminate early in the first year of employment. These homes were not different. Among all leavers, about 45 percent left within the first 3 months, 30 percent more left between the fourth and twelfth month, 20 percent left between the first and third year and 5 percent left after 3 years. One home lost 62 percent of their leavers during the first 3 months. Obviously, selection procedures, orientation and supervision of new employees must be quite different from homes where only 28 percent left during the same period.

SUPPORTIVE INTERVENTIONS

Many administrative interventions were not statistically significant. They neither predicted success nor lack of it, and were found in both groups. They should be thought of as supportive measures and deserve some comment.

SALARIES AND BENEFITS. This variable had to be removed from the study because the length of the study (two years) combined with inflation of course forced all homes to eventually increase salaries. However, at the end of the first year, homes that did nothing but increase salaries either had an increase or no decrease in turnover. Homes that embarked on improved supervisory training, better personnel policies and upgraded supervision of new employees, but did not raise salaries, started to reduce their turnover during the first year.

This further confirms the research that finds that health care employees do not rank money among the top five reasons for staying in a position. Some administrators even conjecture that without any attempt to meet personal and work needs of employees, a pay raise tends to insult the motivations for choosing a health-care position. Those who work principally for money do not tend to gravitate to health care occupations in the first place. This repeated research finding is so frequently disbelieved that it cannot be overemphasized. While salaries and benefits must be competitive, they will not hold employees in a position where other factors are neglected.

PERSONNEL COMMITTEES. Eleven homes either introduced or reactivated employee committees. Three successful and three unsuccessful homes did this. The intervention will be continued by all eleven homes and may be worth considering.

INCREASED RULE ENFORCEMENT. Only 3 homes increased enforcement of rules. This was done where standards of performance were lax and/or not applied uniformly. The home with the greatest change (from 217 to 53 percent) did this because they felt it related directly to turnover. They also decided it related directly to supervisory competence and was incorporated into their supervisory training program. Regular staff commented, "It's about time." "Now we don't have to cope with poor performers." "No one should get by with constant tardiness," etc. The intent of this intervention was not strictness or sternness but fairness and uniformity of standards and handling of problem behaviors.

EXIT INTERVIEWS. Twelve homes increased their information base by seeking reasons for leaving through an exit interview or anonymous questionnaire after termination. All of these homes plan to continue the practice whenever there are changes and in high turnover departments.

ALTERED WORK SCHEDULES. Eight homes altered employee work schedules. This was done by all 3 groups of homes. In some cases it was considered helpful; in others, it was not. The differences were related to the amount of employee participation and monitoring of employee responses before final adoption of a new plan.

HIRED PERSONNEL DIRECTOR. Four homes hired a personnel director. All reported that it freed the administrator and department heads from a great deal of time spent on screening interviews, revising personnel policies and recruitment. None were qualified in the area of HRM.

INCREASED REFERENCE CHECKS. Five homes increased their information on applicants by increasing the number of reference checks. All but one considered it to be useful.

INCREASED ORIENTATION. Eleven homes (3 in the unsuccessful group and 4 in the successful group) increased the length of orientation time. This is deceiving, as it makes a difference whether the time increased from 1 to 2 days or 1 to 5 days. The length of orientation was not significant in any study. One must conclude that the quality and relevance of orientation is not reflected in a specific time frame.

REPLACED NA WITH LPN. Four homes (2 in the successful, 1 in the unsuccessful group) replaced 1 or more nursing assistants with L.P.N.'s. All reported improved quality of care and positive responses from most personnel.

INCREASED EMPLOYEE RECOGNITION. Six homes (3 in the successful and 2 in the unsuccessful group) increased employee recognition. This seems to indicate that other employee relation factors must be in place and that employee recognition, while important, has low impact on turnover.

BUDDY SYSTEM. Two homes in the unsuccessful group used the Buddy system for new employees. Both reported some success with it.

PRIMARY NURSING/NURSING ASSISTANT JOB LEVELS. Six homes (4 in the successful and 1 in the unsuccessful group) initiated primary nursing. All homes reported improved quality of care and plan to continue the system.

INCREASED INSERVICE. Seven homes increased the amount of employee inservice; 1 was in the unsuccessful group and 4 were in the successful group. In fact, 1 in the latter group employed an inservice director for the first time. All homes reported improved care of many residents. Two administrators made the observation that they thought additional inservice gave employees a greater sense of self-worth which was reflected in several subtle ways, such as attitude toward other personnel as well as families.

INCREASED STAFF. Seven homes increased their staffing (4 in the successful and 1 in the unsuccessful group). All homes reported that this had a positive effect on morale, on quality of care and it reduced the amount of tension when one or two persons resigned. Only one administrator indicated that it was too costly. The others felt that it actually decreased their costs.

SUMMARY

In summary, five administrative interventions distinguished the successful from the unsuccessful homes at the statistically significant level. They were:

1. Revised personnel policies.
2. Increased recruitment efforts.
3. Supervisor training program.
4. Avoidance of use of personnel pools.
5. Increased supervision of new employees.

Other interventions, while probably supportive, were not statistically significant. There was no indication that either organizational characteristics or external forces influenced the reduction of turnover in the successful homes. The conclusions of this study should provide optimism for resolving many personnel problems. It indicates that even if turnover is in part influenced by external factors, controlling internal management problems can negate those influences and result in remarkable changes.

REFERENCES

Bales, Jack. "Nursing Centers Take Action to Reduce Employee Turnover," *Cross Reference*, 5:10, November 1975.

Bieter, Margaret S. *The Association Between Employee Dissatisfaction, Turnover and Absenteeism at a Metropolitan Medical Center*, unpublished Master's thesis, Program in Hospital and Health Care Administration, University of Minnesota, 1979.

Boe, Gerald P. "Employee Turnover: Every Supervisor's Problem," *Health Services Manager*, 11 (7):1–2, 1978.

Brayfield, Arthur H. and Crockett, Walter. "Employee Attitudes and Employee Performance," *Psychological Bulletin*, September, 1955.

Brief, Arthur P. "Turnover Among Hospital Nurses: A Suggested Model," *Journal of Nursing Administration*, VI:8, October, 1976.

Burling, Temple, Lentz, Edith, and Wilson, Robert. *The Give and Take in Hospitals*, New York: Putnam Publishing, 1956.

Herzberg, Frederick et al. *Job Attitudes*, Psychological Services of Pittsburgh, Pittsburgh, PA, 1957.

Hickey, T. "In-Service Training in Gerontology," *Gerontologist*, 14:1:57–64, 1974.

Kahne, Merton J. "Suicides in Mental Hospitals: A Study of the Effects of Personnel and Patient Turnover," *Journal of Health and Social Behavior*, 9, 1968.

Kasteler, J. et al. "Personnel Turnover: A Major Problem for Nursing Homes," *Nursing Homes*, Vol. 28, p. 20, January/February 1979.

Mobley, W.H. et al. "Review and Conceptual Analysis of the Employee Turnover Process," *Psychological Bulletin*, 86:3, 493–522, 1979.

Molberg, Elizabeth. *Factors Affecting Nursing Home Nursing Assistants' Intentions of Seeking New Employment*, unpublished Plan B paper, Hubert Humphrey Institute of Public Affairs, University of Minnesota, 1978.

Pecarchik, Robert and Bardin Nelson. "Employee Turnover in Nursing Homes," *American Journal of Nursing*, 73:2:289–90, February 1973.

Pecarchik, R. and Mather, W. "Labor Turnover Cited as Biggest Problem: The Answer May be More Fringe Benefits," *Modern Nursing Home*, 26:43–44, March 1971.

Petersen, Keith. *A Study of Factors Related to Personnel Turnover in Minnesota Hospitals and Nursing Homes*, unpublished Master's thesis, University of Minnesota, 1979.

Price, James L. *The Study of Turnover*, Ames, Iowa: The Iowa State University Press, 1977.

Revans, R.W. *Standards for Morale*, London: Oxford University Press, 1964.

Schwartz, Arthur. "Staff Development and Morale Building in Nursing Homes," *Gerontologist*, 14:1, February 1974.

Schwind, Ann. *Predictions of Representation Election Results in the Health Sector*, Chapter 2 in unpublished Master's thesis, Program in Hospital Care Administration, University of Minnesota, 1978.

Seybolt, John, Pavett, Cynthia, and Walter, Duane. "Turnover Among Nurses: It Can Be Managed," *Journal of Nursing Administration*, VIII: 9:4–9, September, 1978.

Special Committee on Aging, U.S. Senate, *Nursing Home Care in the United States: Failure in Public Policy*, Introductory Report, 1974 and 1975, Supporting Paper No. 4, U.S. Government Printing Office, Washington DC.

Vroom, Victor. *Work and Motivation*, New York: John Wiley & Sons, 1964.

Chapter 10

RECRUITMENT, SCREENING AND SELECTION OF PERSONNEL

Ruth Stryker

Recruitment, screening, and selection efforts have been shown to be the major steps in attracting and obtaining the right persons for your positions. This involves putting to use many of the suggestions which originate from research and well established personnel practices.

RECRUITMENT

The purpose of recruitment is to give you choices in filling your positions. Recruitment is important, but it is not related to retention. Unless an organization provides a support system, recruitment will be a never-ending cost with no payoffs. It can be compared to running water into a bathtub with an open drain. You can never fill the tub unless you have some mechanism to hold the water. An organization must be able to both attract and retain desirable employees. Recruitment, however, is a first step.

The number of recruitment methods is endless. Newspaper ads, bonuses, public service teas, church contacts, community signs, former employees, present employees, announcements, families, local schools and employment agencies are commonly used. A brief comment on a few of these methods seems warranted.

First of all, a satisfied employee, former employees, and affiliating students are your best available recruiters. One gains a reputation as a good employer from these persons, not from disgruntled and unhappy persons who have left the organization. Employees and former employees are not neutral. They either enhance the image of your organization as a good employer or discourage every potential employee (and client also) they meet.

This consideration suggests an often forgotten recruitment method;

namely, transfer and promotion. Does a nursing assistant want to be a dietary aide or vice versa? Would the maid on 2 East be a good housekeeping director? Posting all job openings in the organization is frequently fruitful, as lateral moves may be desired by some employees.

Newspaper ads, unless you are the only home in a community, must highlight some special or worthwhile aspect of the job or the organization. For instance, what does, "Wanted: Nursing Assistants, all shifts," convey to a reader? It tells me that this organization has a lot of openings and I wonder why. Second, it does not state any personal or education requirements, so I wonder what if any, there are. It also looks like a lot of other ads. The more thoughtful applicant, the one you want, is going to search for an ad that mentions some interest in its employees and/or some standards of care. Ad 1 invites applicants who do not care about such things.

Administrators should read the Want Ads in order to compare themselves with their competitors and learn how to capitalize on the assets of their own organization. Here are two examples taken from a Sunday newspaper.

> AD 1—   RN'S LPN'S
>   Part time, full time, 7–3, 3–11 shifts.
>   Contact Jane Jones, Mon–Fri 8–4. EOE
>   Lake Hill Nursing Home 438-1218.

> AD 2—NURSES WHO WANT TO GET INVOLVED
>   Tired of tubes, bottles and machinery?
>   Why not become a geriatric nurse?
>   The Community Nursing Home takes
>   pride in its personalized care and its
>   geriatric rehabilitation education
>   program. We offer competitive
>   salaries, flexible scheduling and
>   a new opportunity to practice
>   your profession more independently.
>   Call Mary Johnson, 436-8121, for an
>   appointment at your convenience. EOE

The author happened to know the administrators of both homes and called to inquire about the response to the ads. Lake Hill received only one call from an L.P.N. The Community home received calls from six R.N.'s and seventeen L.P.N.'s! While their ad was more expensive, it paid off. They understood their "specialness," tried to locate disenchanted hospital nurses, and offered training, flexible scheduling and competitive salaries. They had a target, and it did not invite just anyone.

Knowing what long-term care nurses like about their jobs can assist in identifying nurses for long-term care. According to Kaye White, job satisfaction comes from: (1) greater autonomy in decisions regarding delivery of care, (2) closer relationships with residents and families, (3) more opportunities to use professional and administrative skills, (4) time to talk to and understand patients, (5) seeing the results of well-planned team care plans, (6) use of a greater variety of skills including teaching, and (7) less organizational bureaucracy than hospitals. Some of the stresses of the job relate to (1) death and dying, (2) communication problems with residents, (3) emotional commitment as a family surrogate and (4) difficulty in separating work concerns from one's personal life. Seeking nurses who like the autonomy and responsibilities of a nursing home position and helping them to deal with the stresses that go along with the position will certainly encourage them to stay and continue to feel challenged.

Too frequent advertising, inappropriate timing and other factors may actually do an organization more harm than good. Timing may be important. September and January are considered good recruiting months by some health care providers. Such differences may vary among communities and should be observed on an individual basis.

If you know your turnover cycles (one reason for monitoring turnover quarterly), you can plan ahead for recruiting new staff. Waiting for a predictable resignation pressures an employer to accept questionable applicants. Recruiting for predictable vacancies in advance is no more costly and gives you a chance to choose from a greater number of applicants.

Bonuses to employees for locating a new employee may backfire. First, a bonus tells the world that you are desperate. This could be due to a 2 percent unemployment rate in your area or because your home has a bad reputation. In either instance, a bonus game among employees may develop, leaving you where you were, but after considerable expense.

Other good recruiting methods include neighborhood teas for potential applicants, using the home as a site for a geriatric nurse refresher course and inviting nurses from the community to your inservice programs. Your reputation as an employer and the way your adjacent community perceives your organization is particularly important in rural areas and blue collar neighborhoods in metropolitan areas.

Families can be another ally in recruitment. One nursing home formally called in families to explain the problem of short staffing. Within a month, they had three new R.N.'s, two L.P.N.'s and seven nursing assistants. Again, this assumes that you are giving good care to residents. This obviously will not work if families have their relatives on the waiting list of another home.

Some homes find that they benefit over a period of time when they serve as a training site for nursing schools, vocational schools, training dietary workers and others. This can have a positive impact if the training is made challenging **and** the students like the organization. If a nursing home allows itself to be a training site for routinized custodial care, it is unlikely to gain employees in the end. On the other hand, these persons will look to you for employment if they found some challenges, learned to care for the elderly and found personnel working well together.

The demography of potential employees is changing just as it is for the elderly. School closings due to smaller numbers of school children translates to fewer part time students in the labor pool. It will be incumbent upon nursing homes to look to other age-groups such as the middle-aged woman whose children are in college, some of the young old (sixty-five to seventy-five years of age) themselves and more flexible working hours for women with children still at home.

In summary, recruitment efforts should indicate both an interest in the potential employee and a concern for residents. The ideal goal is of course to recruit more applicants than you need so that you have choices. Even when you do not have this luxury, screening the recruit or drop-in applicant is needed to prevent the acquisition of persons who may do more harm than going short-handed.

SCREENING

Employers either distort or disregard the employment process when they talk about "recruiting employees." One recruits **applicants.** Within a group of applicants, you may or may not find an employee you want. If you recruit employees (employ anyone who comes to your door), it is almost predictable that you will not only have high turnover, but absenteeism, low morale among employees and poor quality of patient care as well.

Let us examine this concept a little further. Two of the high turnover homes in our study reported at least eight to ten "no show" or "no call" terminations every quarter. Both homes also had a very high absentee rate. This meant that remaining staff was unexpectedly left shorthanded repeatedly every month. Desperation employment of high risk persons followed and the cycle was never broken. This has insidious effects on other employees. They may feel it reflects on the worth of their work (the organization would not do this if their work was thought to be important). Employees become both physically and emotionally exhausted from carrying extra work loads or working extra shifts and it results in increased absenteeism and/or sick time. This nurtures high turnover. The effect on residents must also be very depressing.

Some administrators screen unskilled workers but will immediately hire any R.N., L.P.N., R.P.T. or other professional, assuming that their education and/or license makes them suitable job candidates. This fallacy leads to still different problems. Because such persons must assume supervisory positions and direct programs, it is imperative that they do not have a personality disorder and that they either have geriatric knowledge or are willing to learn. In other words, the first step in reducing turnover is to try to recruit applicants, not employees. You then screen the applicants, a process of filtering out undesirable candidates and keeping desirable ones. It helps to prevent employing the wrong persons, which only amounts to a temporary body count anyway.

Some administrators will argue that they cannot do this as they will receive a deficiency and/or fine from the health department because they may go below the required hours of care per patient. An administrator must deal with this or turnover problems will be hopelessly locked into the organization. First of all, an organization can hire above the minimum requirements in order to catch up on training and increase the confidence of employees and residents, in order to begin to break the turnover cycle. Secondly, the organization can document its recruiting and screening efforts. Some health department surveyors currently accept this as evidence of effort to increase staff and realize that a short staff may be preferable to a staff of inappropriate short stay or no show workers. Nursing home organizations should work with local officials to help them to understand this dynamic and to make the surveyor decision on this issue more uniform.

So much for the importance of screening applicants. What are some of the steps?

THE APPLICATION BLANK: Traditionally, the application form has been viewed as a screening device, rightly or wrongly. The application form will probably not predict tenure, but it will give you some basic information on which to build. It is imperative that your application form does not violate fair employment practice standards (see Appendix A, Guidelines for a Nondiscriminatory Application Form).

Barbara Portnoy studied the applications of 311 nursing, dietary, and housekeeping assistants, employed by the three long-term care organizations where she was the executive administrator. The purpose of the study was to determine if certain items of the application form could predict whether an employee would have short or long tenure. This exhaustive piece of research concluded that this was impossible. However, reflection upon her lack of findings led to some startling conclusions and recommendations for managers. Some of Portnoy's findings and suggestions are as follows:

1. Supervisors and administrators employ persons on the basis of characteristics they **believe** to be associated with tenure, such as previous health care experience, personal references, tenure on previous jobs, graduation from high school, distance from job, etc. Since none of these were associated with tenure, new criteria for selection must replace these false assumptions. Indeed, previous health care experience and distance from employment were inversely related to tenure at one of her organizations!

2. Employee exit interview information should be studied in depth.

3. All management staff should review and select organizational and job information to be given to applicants so that actual work is portrayed accurately. Both monetary and nonfinancial rewards should be included. This will lessen misunderstandings before, rather than after, employment.

4. Application forms should be clear and understandable to the least educated applicants.

5. Interviewers should be more diligent in pursuing omitted questions and incomplete or ambiguous responses on the application blank. In fact, one nursing home discovered that most of their short stay employees gave incomplete work histories and vague answers when questioned about these items.

CHECKING REFERENCES: Obtaining an honest work reference is becoming more and more difficult. However, it is worth appropriate efforts. A written release of information by an employee may be possible. Certainly a telephone call to verify if employment and the dates did in fact occur is in order. Sometimes a question such as "Would you rehire?" will be answered. Other desirable questions include: Was this person's work above or below average in terms of amount and quality? What were his or her strengths and weaknesses? Was there a problem with attendance, interpersonal relations or work performance? Why did he or she leave? You may not obtain all you want, but some information is better than none. At the minimum, you will have verified a previous job.

Checking personal references is usually nonproductive unless you are also acquainted with someone listed. Success or failure in a previous job may predict the same result in your organization. However, there are exceptions, and talking to the potential employee about an unsuccessful job experience may elicit information that would not be relevant in your situation.

In summary, turnover can be prevented by screening out undesirable persons with a history of job hopping and unsatisfactory work. Screening recruits may also be the first step of a quality assurance program.

INTERVIEWING: Entire books have been written on interviewing. Administrators and department heads must learn interviewing skills. This should include learning the distinction between direct and nondirect methods, subjective and objective information, reading and sending nonverbal and verbal messages, dealing with one's own prejudices, generalizing from one characteristic, legal implications of some questions, preparing for, conducting and terminating the interview, improved listening skills, etc. In addition to obtaining information about the applicant, the applicant will need to know about the job—the hours, the pay, the nonmonetary satisfactions, etc. The applicant should also see the job description.

There are a few special areas of concern for long-term care organizations. They should be dealt with in openness initially. Why does the individual want to work with the elderly? How did or do they feel about their parents and grandparents? It is important that they realize that older people are just like any other age-group. Some are more likable than others and some are more difficult to get along with than others.

Interviews should try to explore certain attitudes and feelings that relate to the clientele. If the clientele is aged, one might want to explore some of the following questions:

> Do you have an interest in a relationship that will last for a prolonged period?
> How uncomfortable do you feel in the presence of mentally and physically disabled persons? Note: You do not want employees who are

uncomfortable with their own aging, who wish to have people depend on them, or have patronizing or infantalizing attitudes.

Do you believe that most elderly have a rehabilitation potential, at least to some degree?

Tell me about the older relatives or friends you have known. This might elicit feelings of affection, hostility and/or realism. Usually, it is only when someone is unconscious of anger or fear of parental authority that there is a potential danger of acting out such feelings with residents.

Do you feel you know yourself well enough not to act blindly if a resident reminded you of someone you disliked?

Have you ever experienced the death of a close relative or friend?

What did you like best and least in your previous job?

If the applicant is a professional, you might ask, "To what extent do you think that the typical professional role interferes with a resident's needs?"

Several organizations have developed small cases regarding events in a nursing home. The applicant responds to the interviewer and discusses the cases. These responses are also used to assess applicants. Both applicants and interviewers report very favorable responses to this method.

Some research has shown that turnover is high when the employee and the employer differ in job expectations. Therefore, it is important to mention some of the special features of long-term care. Then, if it is not what the applicant expected, he or she can reject the job **prior** to employment. Factors that fall into this area include such things as the following:

Long-term involvement with residents can sometimes become emotionally draining when a favorite resident becomes ill and dies.

The role of an employee is often that of a friend, especially for a resident with few friends or family living at a distance.

The role of an employee is to help the resident stay as independent as possible. The long-term care organization does not need or want employees who obtain their satisfactions by feeling superior to the infirm, by fostering dependence or by infantalizing the confused.

The interview is not considered a very accurate way of assessing a potential employee. Because of this, it is often wise to have two persons interview (separately) an applicant. Each person is likely to see different strengths and weaknesses and you are likely to assess the applicant with greater accuracy. Certainly, one of the interviewers should be the department head.

An interview can also assess inservice and training needs for an individual. For instance, a nice young college freshman would like to work three evenings a week for at least two years. She likes older people and has been close to a widowed grandmother. She is also going to become a social worker. She has never experienced the death of a close friend or relative and has never read anything about bereavement or care of a dying person. If you hire this young woman, you would want the inservice director to give her some readings in this area and make sure that she attended any inservice classes on this subject. She would then be less uncomfortable about her skills when such a situation occurs.

In summary, the interview should include a discussion of the job itself, the various tasks involved, the salary, and the many personal ramifications of the job. This will help to make the interview as predictive as possible. Discussing these things prior to employment sets the tone and expectations of the job initially. If the applicant is later employed, there will be better congruence or agreement about job expectations. Those who did not agree with or like your stated expectations will most likely not agree to work for you. Thus, you will prevent many poor matches.

Tour: Every interview should include a tour of the work area under consideration, an introduction to any coworkers on duty and an introduction to one or more residents. A potential employee cannot envision his or her work from an office. The sights and sounds of the nursing home must be viewed first hand before an applicant is in a position to decide to work there.

The DeKalb County Nursing Home reports that residents participate in this process (Bahr). Volunteer residents have some briefing on interviewing and take applicants on a tour of the home. They observe the person's reaction to the disabled, the helpless and the disoriented. They watch for nonverbal communications such as acceptance, boredom, interest, etc. Besides the positive benefit of having another opinion and observation of an applicant, it provides a perspective that supervisory personnel could not judge from their conversation. While an applicant may say he/she likes older people, this method provides a sort of pre-test for behavioral responses. This home reports that new employees express appreciation for meeting residents prior to employment and residents of course feel very positively about being a part of the employment process.

SELECTION

According to Longest and Clawson, "there is good reason to believe that perhaps the single most important factor in reducing personnel turnover is careful selection of employees." If this is true, then the final decision to hire should be made by the immediate department head. This person knows best the job requirements, the personalities of present employees and the dynamics of the work environment. For this reason, the department head has the most insight into the total situation. In addition, this helps to develop a sense of responsibility and accountability for his or her department.

The selection process is the assembling of all available information about an applicant, the assessment of this information and the decision to employ or not to employ one individual among several applicants. It is crucial that all steps be followed if management is serious about its mission. This of course does not mean that you will have no doubts about the person you hire. Selection is always an act of faith. However, you will know what those doubts are and you will be prepared to deal with them if they present themselves. In other words, you will know ahead of time what inservice areas of assistance that may be warranted.

You are ready to select an employee for employment if:

All federal and state guidelines are met.
The application form is complete and checked for completion and accuracy.
The interviewer(s) has been trained.
The trained interviewer feels that the applicant should be assigned to a particular job (not any job).
The interviewee has seen the job description, knows what hours s/he will be assigned, wages to expect, visited the work area and met some peers as well as residents.
License of professional persons verified.
Reference checks have been attempted and preferably received by letter or telephone.
The applicant does not have a high turnover profile (under twenty-five years of age, single, history of job hopping, such as more than three or four jobs in the past five years), does not have transportation difficulty, only needs temporary employment or possesses inappropriate skills, etc.

Employers in health care often overlook one very important concept in the selection process. People are more likely to stay challenged and interested in a position if they can work at their **higher** levels of ability. Working at one's lowest capability soon results in boredom and lack of interest. Therefore, the selection process should attempt to match the person's ability as well as interest on the job. If a job requires repetitious tasks and dependability rather than analysis and judgment about changing situations, a borderline retarded person might be the ideal employee. Professional persons would, on the other hand, be allowed to use the widest, not the narrowest, range of judgment for which he or she is educated. In other words, employing a person who has education and ambition beyond which the job can offer, incurs risk of early turnover.

If you tend to want to hire someone who has more than one dubious recommendation, a reminder not to hire someone else's rejects is in order. However, if there is only one such situation, it is wise to pursue the matter with the applicant to see if there is a plausible reason for a poor recommendation in the past. After all, there are bad employers, just as there are bad employees, and most of us have experienced both sides of such a situation. If you are satisfied with the explanation about a particular job, it is not out of order to employ the person.

There is one other important consideration when administrators and department heads are selecting persons who will give direct care to residents. It relates to attitudes. An untrained person with positive attitudes toward a particular clientele, especially the disabled and the elderly, often has a more therapeutic effect than a trained person with a negative attitude. The latter may actually cause increased fear or psychological withdrawal by patients. It is far easier to teach technical skills than to change attitudes. At this juncture, it is important to point out the license to practice a particular profession does not guarantee positive motivations for dealing with a particular clientele. In other words, knowledge and skill is important, but attitudes can either dilute or strengthen those skills.

The final point in selection is to prepare an initial plan of orientation for the individual. This is best done with the individual and can be explored during the interview, discussed in a letter or telephone call when the position is offered, or it can be developed in greater depth on the first day on the job. It of course may need revision during the first few weeks of employment.

SUMMARY

Recruiting, screening and selection efforts will have many benefits. Not only will they reduce turnover, but they will improve organizational function. First, you will have reduced the number of gross misfits entering your organization. This in turn will reduce the number of persons needing to be discharged. Second, by giving the employee a chance to learn about the job, applicants will have greater information on which to base their decision to accept or reject the position. Those who are unsuited for the job are more likely to reject it before going on the payroll. This is far preferable to having someone come to work and then not show up or quit during the first days or weeks of employment. Thus, you will be spared the financial cost of nonproductive work and wasted teaching time. Third, other personnel will be spared a great deal of unexpected and erratic work requirements caused by having such persons on staff. Fourth, residents and patients will not be subjected to inept, uncaring or fearful employees. Lastly, you will have set standards and expectations upon which you can build new employees. This will give present employees a sense of confidence in management and will give residents a sense of confidence that you do not wish to subject them to inappropriate care givers.

In other words, a new employee will not attach much importance to the job unless the organization does. Present employees will not respect the organization unless the organization demonstrates respect for their working conditions. Residents will be better able to maintain their self-respect if they are not forced to deal with preventable changes and disruptions in their environment.

REFERENCES

Bahr, Janet, "Residents Participate in Selection of New Employees," *Journal of Gerontological Nursing,* 6:1:43, January, 1980.

Longest, B.B. and Clawson, D.E., "The Effect of Selected Factors on Hospital Turnover Rates," *Personnel Journal,* pp. 30–34, January 1974.

Portnoy, Barbara, *A Study of the Usefulness of Employee Application Items in Predicting Tenure,* unpublished master's thesis, University of Minnesota, 1979.

White, Kaye, "Nurse Recruitment and Retention in Long-Term Care," *Journal of Long-Term Care Administrators,* VIII:3:25–36, Fall 1980.

Chapter 11

PERSONNEL POLICIES WITH SPECIAL IMPACT ON EMPLOYEES

Ruth Stryker

GENERAL COMMENTS

Personnel policies and procedures reflect the concern of management for its workers and influence the success of many organizational goals. Certain policies are especially helpful in producing a positive corporate culture.

Perhaps the best way to view the importance of the content of this chapter is through Herzberg's two-factor theory. He calls these Motivation and Hygiene factors. He describes adequate and appropriate wage and personnel policies as positive "hygiene factors." They are important to the work climate, but they do not motivate. He goes on to say, however, that if wages and policies are inadequate and unfair, they cause job dissatisfaction. The removal of such dissatisfiers, however, does not create job satisfaction. The removal of these dissatisfiers merely makes a more "hygienic" work environment.

Once an organization has fair and adequate wage and personnel policies, it can go on with the business of job satisfaction. Job satisfaction involves motivation which in turn encompasses the nature of the tasks performed and opportunities for achievement. This chapter concerns improving the general hygiene of the work environment by removing dissatisfiers. It will include (1) definitions to differentiate policies, procedures and rules, (2) guidelines for writing policies and procedures, and (3) suggestions for content of personnel policies that have been selected because of their special impact on personnel.

The existence or nonexistence of certain policy content and its wording warrant the scrutiny of the administrator. Some policies should be removed from an organization's policy book because they pertain to either a bygone social era or outdated circumstances. For example, one administrator found a policy on employee meal hours which stated that all employees had to eat at either 11:00 AM or 11:30 AM in order for kitchen help to serve patient meals by 12:15 PM. However, for five years they had been serving employee meals cafeteria style from their expanded kitchen between 11:00 AM and 1:00 PM. This kind of situation makes a joke of policy books and deters personnel from using them or being able to rely on them.

Outdated policies are one problem. Unwritten policies are still a different problem. Sometimes things are done, but no one knows just why, nor can they be found in writing. Unwritten policies especially confuse new employees because situations are handled differently and inconsistently by supervisors. Lack of uniform standards and expectations of course make employees anxious. This was evident at one nursing home where nursing assistants complained that evening charge nurses expected different things of them. One evening charge nurse required that fresh water be given to residents at meal time. Another insisted that it be given after meals and at bedtime, and a third did not allow residents to have any water at the bedside after 8:00 PM because there were fewer calls for assistance to the bathroom at night. The nursing assistants complained about these different expectations and expressed their disappointment that only one of the charge nurses seemed to be more concerned about fluid intake than work for the night nurses. This situation required a written policy—in this case, one that benefitted resident care.

In some instances, a written policy may be perfectly adequate, but implemented only on whim or by certain individuals. All of the above situations reduce the effectiveness of policies, decrease respect for management personnel and cause conflict between personnel.

The actual content of a policy or procedure may cause problems and frequently explains inconsistent implementation. If a policy interferes with day to day supervision or causes frequent frustration for either employees or supervisors, it needs to be analyzed and reviewed with the staff whom it affects and then changed accordingly.

Finally, the wording of policies is crucial. They must be clear and concise in order for the reader to understand the intent. Wordiness and imprecise words can easily result in unclear meanings and a variety of interpretations. The way a policy is stated is also important. Because health care organizations have historical roots from both the church and the military, there is a frequent tendency to make dogmatic statements that sound very much like military orders. Administrators and supervisors should select their language carefully in order to guard against this pitfall because it can produce both resistance and resentment on the part of personnel.

While all personnel policies and procedures have a collective influence on personnel, certain ones are particularly important and may even provide grist for union organizing in some cases. In fact, one segment of the literature suggests that poor institutional personnel policies and practices (which reflect its pattern of employee relations), is the single most important determinant of attracting unions. The same discontent that makes some employees seek unionization of course makes other employees leave an organization. The following policies have been selected for discussion because of the strong influence of these issues: paid time away from work (holidays, vacation and sick leave), disciplinary measures, handling grievances, employee assistance programs, compensation and work schedules.

DEFINITIONS

Before we discuss these policies, it is important to define our terms. All too frequently, a policy is confused with a rule, a procedure or a regulation. The following definitions will help the reader to think through the differences:

DIRECTIVE. A directive describes a specific course of action for a one-time event. For instance when a patient unit closes for some reason, a directive is required to establish a system for moving patients and supplies.

Directives are misused when they describe new rules, policies or procedures for repeated use. They are then lost and rarely incorporated into the general policy manual.

RULE. A rule describes a required course of action in a given situation. Rules do not allow for individual judgment. "No smoking" in certain areas or in the presence of oxygen are examples. Because of the rigidity of rules, it is best to use them only when necessary and to have as few as possible.

REGULATION. A regulation describes a course of action required by law.

PROCEDURE. A procedure describes the steps in performing a task.

Filling out organizational forms and performing passive range of motion exercises are examples.

POLICY. A policy describes a recommended course of action for carrying out an organizational goal.

"Recommended" is the key word in this definition. A policy allows for individual judgment in determining the appropriateness and method of an action in different situations. In general, the purposes of policies are to (1) convey the thinking of management in order to assist middle management and other employees in their daily activities, (2) express and guide the implementation of organizational goals and (3) provide information and reference material for employees.

In practice, however, most policies have both guidelines for action and some rules. As you read the following policies try to identify the rules imbedded in each policy, so that you understand which statements allow for flexibility and those that do not.

FORMAT FOR WRITING POLICIES

When policies are written, they need to have a consistent and easily readable format. Generous use of headings and subheadings are important for easy reference, especially for someone who merely wants to look up one part of a policy or just the procedure for carrying it out.

Title

The title should describe the subject of the policy as clearly as possible. For example, a policy entitled Passing Water could mean passing drinking water to patients, or it could mean helping paraplegics to pass urine while on a bladder training program. In one organization, the policy entitled Passing Water meant the latter. This kind of surprise content is found more frequently than one would like to think.

Purpose

Every policy should begin with a purpose. This has several functions. First, it forces the management of an organization to think through why a policy exists. Is it needed at all? If things are done "just because it says so," there may be less enthusiasm for carrying it out. It also helps administration to evaluate each policy to see if it actually carries out its purpose.

Secondly, it provides a mind set for the reader before he or she starts to read the policy. It provides some understanding of the thinking behind it and will seem a more reasonable thing to do. The stated purpose should reflect administration's beliefs and position on a particular subject.

Third, policies should rarely result from single person or situation incidents. An outside reader can identify these because they were so obviously developed in lieu of counseling an individual staff member in a particular situation. Policies should guide behavior for all employees. If it is developed because one employee or one supervisor did not do this, it can insult other employees.

Policy

There are usually multiple facets to a policy. In other words, there are sub-policies to an overall policy and they usually cluster around several aspects of the policy. This is handled by the use of headings. Organizing ideas under headings is illustrated in some of the sample policies on the following pages.

Procedure

Many policies stand alone and have no accompanying procedure. For example, there may be a policy that all employees use the parking lot in the rear of the building. There is no need for a procedure. However, if a policy requires all employees to use a time clock, a procedure may be needed to tell employees what to do if they make a mistake, forget to punch in and out or become ill at work. This author recommends that if a procedure relates directly to a policy, it should accompany that policy rather than place it in a separate Procedure Book.

SOME SAMPLE POLICIES

Paid Time Away From Work

Time away from work is paid by an organization when employees take vacation, holiday and sick time. Vacation and holiday time can be scheduled, but sick time usually comes up unexpectedly and is rarely scheduled. In addition, most organizations find, or at least suspect, that sick time is frequently abused by one or two day absences which are taken to fulfill personal or psychological needs. While this may arise from legitimate needs, personnel policies often leave employees no other option but to call in sick when fatigue, the need for personal time or family pressures accumulate. First, rather typical policies for paid time away from work will be described. Second, several alternative policies will be described. The latter are sometimes called "employee incentive time" policies which have been developed to reduce unscheduled and unexpected absenteeism.

Sick Leave

I. Purpose: To enable employees to receive pay when away from work due to accident or illness.
II. Policy:
    A. A six-month period of employment is required before sick-leave benefits will be paid.
    B. Sick leave benefits are accumulated as follows:
        1. Full time employees (forty hours/week)—one day a month up to a maximum of thirty days.
        2. Part time employees (thirty-nine or fewer hours/week)—percent of time worked based on 173 hours/month will be the percent of eight hours of sick leave earned per month up to a maximum of twenty days. Example: Employee works 100 hours in month (58% of 173 hours). Employee earns four and one half hours sick leave (58% of eight hours) for that month of 100 hours of work.
    C. A statement by a physician or nurse practitioner will be required:
        1. When brief illnesses occur monthly.
        2. To verify ability to return to work after an extended illness.
III. Procedure:
    A. In case of illness, the supervisor must be notified as far in advance as possible.
    B. Upon return to work:
        1. Present letter from M.D. or N.P. if this has been requested.
        2. Mark "ill" for each day you were off on your time card.

It should be noted that some organizations do not pay for one, two or three day absences in order to discourage their frequency. It may do this, but it also penalizes someone who gets a migraine headache or twenty-four hour flu and tends to encourage some employees to come to work when they might spread colds or flu. In addition, it penalizes conscientious workers who do not use sick days indiscriminately.

**Alternative Methods of Handling
Sick Time and Vacation Time**

Several systems have been initiated to encourage employees to use sick leave more discriminately and to reduce one and two day absences. Before starting such a program, it is critical to calculate the cost of absenteeism and sick leave (the cost paid to sick employees plus the cost of replacing the sick employee, added overtime or the use of an employment agency). Then a new system can be evaluated accurately when it is initiated. One hospital did just that. Its absentee rate went from 3.9 percent to 2.1 percent in one year. They estimated that this saved about $34,000. The cost of their innovative policy was $30,000 compared to an estimated cost of $64,000, had their former sick leave policy remained in effect.

Muscatine General Hospital in Muscatine, Iowa developed a plan for paid leave that combines holiday, vacation and sick leave time. This will serve as an excellent example. Each employee accumulates a bank of paid leave time which enables employees to choose how and when they use their time. The policy is considered highly successful and is adapted with their permission.

DEFINITION. Paid Leave is a fund of hours, earned by employees that allows them to choose how to use their paid time off. However, if sick or absent on a holiday, or on a day before or after a holiday, pay may be forfeited.

BASIS FOR EARNED TIME. Each full-time employee will earn Paid Leave hours based upon the years of full-time service (2080 hours per year). The number of earned Paid Leave hours per pay period depends upon the length of service at the hospital.

Years of Service	% of an hour earned for each hour worked
Employment thru 4th year	6.625%
Employment 5th thru 9th year	7.375%
Employment 10th thru 14th year	8.500%
Employment 15th year or longer	9.652%

Payment of Paid Leave is computed at straight time hourly rate of pay, without regard to shift differential, overtime, call pay, etc.

Paid Leave will become available for use after six months of employment.

HOLIDAYS.

1. Eight hours of Paid Leave will be added to each full-time employee's Paid Leave fund during the pay period in which the holiday occurs. Paid Leave will become available to full-time employees as the holidays occur, provided the employee has worked at least forty hours from date of employment until the day of the holiday.

2. The seven recognized holidays are:

   New Year's Day
   Memorial Day
   July 4th
   Labor Day
   Thanksgiving
   Christmas
   Employee's Birthday

3. Terminating employees must work on or after the holiday to be eligible to receive this holiday component. Part-time employees will earn the regular percentage of Paid Leave for their hours worked.

4. The recognized holiday consists of a twenty-four hour period beginning at midnight on the eve of the holiday and ending at midnight of the holiday itself. The work shifts to be included in the holiday shall be those in which a majority of the time worked falls within the hours of the holiday.

5. Employees of departments which are closed on the holiday are expected to take that day off. If the department is not closed, and the employee wishes to take Paid Leave for the holiday, it must be applied for in advance. Approval of the request as well as the scheduling of holiday hours are at the discretion of the department head or supervisor.

REQUESTING LEAVE. Paid Leave will be granted upon request whenever possible. Preference is given to those with the longest service, provided the employee has been employed for at least six months and the request is submitted to the Department Head in accordance with departmental policy.

ACCUMULATING PAID LEAVE. Paid Leave hours can be accumulated up to a maximum of 480 hours (60 days). No additional hours will be added beyond that total.

PAID LEAVE AND ILLNESS. (1) Paid Leave is used when an employee is ill for one or more days. (2) Paid Leave may not be used for illness prior to the completion of six months of employment. (3) When ill, an employee must notify the Supervisor or Department Head as soon as possible and state the nature of the illness.

PAID LEAVE AND TERMINATION. (1) Payment will not be made in lieu of taking Paid Leave time except in case of termination. In this instance, payment will be made for any unused Paid Leave earned up to and including the last day actually worked. This payment will be made as a lump sum and included in the paycheck for the last pay period actually worked. (2) If termination occurs prior to six months of employment, no Paid Leave hours will be paid. (3) No Paid Leave will be paid when the hospital terminates the employee. (4) If an employee is absent for three consecutively scheduled work days without notifying the Supervisor, employment will be terminated. Accrued and otherwise earned Paid Leave hours will not be paid under these circumstances. (5) Any employee suspended without pay for disciplinary reasons may not use Paid Leave hours during the time of suspension.

PAYMENT OF PAID LEAVE.

1. The hospital will not advance Paid Leave beyond that which has been earned.
2. Employees who wish to have Leave pay included in paychecks in advance of a vacation, should make this request to the Department Head at least one week before pay day.

Grievances

Most personnel directors agree that an ideal grievance policy probably does not exist. There are two principal reasons for this. First, no grievance policy can possibly anticipate the great variety of gripes, conflicts, complaints and offended feelings that are usually lumped under the rubric, grievances. In addition to the policy itself and the nature of a grievance, the attitude of those implementing the policy strongly influences the outcome. In spite of these problems, it is essential to have some mechanism for both surfacing and resolving employee problems.

Not having a grievance policy can merely provide another reason for someone to join the ranks of terminating employees. This is corroborated in a study of eleven hospitals in Atlanta by Longest and Clawson.

They found that whether or not there was a written grievance policy had a strong influence on turnover. It is also known that when organizational discontent is exhibited by turnover, **and** there is no way of airing conflicts, union organizing is a distinct possibility.

The purpose of a grievance policy is to provide a formalized method of upward communication of a problem. If a lower level of management blocks or does not resolve a problem, it allows review of the matter by persons who are further removed from the immediate situation. The following policy and procedure is one way of accomplishing this.

Grievance Policy

I. Purpose: To provide a mechanism for resolving problems and misunderstandings between management and employees in a fair and equitable manner.

II. Policy: Each employee shall be afforded the opportunity to express grievances without fear of retribution or termination. If the employee does not feel that the problem has been resolved to his/her satisfaction, he/she shall have the opportunity to request that it be presented to a higher level of management.

III. Procedure:

A. Grievances should first be discussed with the immediate supervisor.

*B. If the immediate supervisor does not resolve the grievance to the employee's satisfaction within five days, the employee may direct the grievance in writing to the administrator.

C. After receiving the written grievance, the administrator shall meet in person with the employee and the supervisor together or individually, and present a written decision to the employee and the supervisor within five days.

D. If the employee is still not satisfied, he/she may present the issue to the Grievance Committee, which will be composed of:
one board member
one employee representative selected by employees
one person selected by the person presenting the grievance
one department head selected by the department head involved.

---

*In larger institutions, there may be other levels of redress, such as the department head or personnel director, before it is taken to the Administrator.

E. The Grievance Committee's decision shall be final.

WAGES AND BENEFITS

While it has been clearly demonstrated that people do not rate money as their primary incentive for work, especially in health care occupations, salary and/or wages can obviously deter or encourage workers. High pay rarely holds someone in an unsatisfactory work situation or job, just as low pay rarely causes someone to quit who is well satisfied. Again, this is just one of many factors to be considered in trying to maintain a stable staff.

Compensation management should be studied elsewhere. However, it would be remiss not to discuss a few guidelines that relate pay to attracting qualified personnel.

First of all, administrators must carefully review their wage and salary schedules and benefit packages. The following questions are basic to beginning such a review:

1. How many positions in my organization begin at the minimum rate required by law? Since this is also required of all competitors, it should be examined in terms of any position that is difficult to fill. Entry wages may be an obstacle.

2. How many positions are currently open? Is this fairly usual? Are the same positions usually open? If the number and kind of job openings are fairly constant, the wage and salary structure should be examined.

3. How does this organization compare to similar organizations in the community? Do wages contribute to the reasons for resignations? Every health care organization must stay informed of how its pay scales compare with comparable jobs and similar organizations in the community. The Employment Office in most states provides regional data that describes salary ranges for major occupational groups. Many organizations do their own surveys, either formally or informally, and some professional associations have such information available.

One large nursing home regularly had about 90 openings among 400 positions. This situation mitigated against a stable work force, locating competent staff and the ability to provide quality of care. After considerable study, the organization discovered its starting salaries were in the lowest quartile in that community for similar positions.

In another instance, an administrator attempted to justify noncompetitive wage scales by saying, "If they just work for money, then we don't want them." His lack of understanding of employee motivation and competitive job opportunities perpetuates a chronic staff shortage. First of all, health care organizations are indeed lucky. If most of their employees "just worked for money," they would have to close down. Second, research in this area clearly reveals that health care workers place money about sixth or seventh among their reasons for staying in a job. In large metropolitan areas, applicants can usually choose between several very fine organizations. One could hardly expect a potential employee to select the lowest paying organization for an employer. If an organization becomes complacent because of its philosophy and goals, it will lose good employees and thus strengthen one's competitors.

4. Is the wage structure designed to encourage tenure? If an employee likes a job, he or she is more likely to leave if the top of the pay scale is reached in two or three years. A minimum and maximum wage level for each job level is essential. The range between the two must be wide enough to provide some incentive for an employee to stay. Some organizations have as much as a 30 percent range between minimum and maximum salaries.

The timing of wage increases must be spread over a period of years. Some organizations give rather substantial raises during the first year, then taper off rather drastically and sometimes even stop after three or four years. The Paid Leave policy of Muscatine General Hospital previously described has taken up to fifteen years of employment into account. In addition, most experts recommend that the increases become greater toward the end of the time frame rather than early in the schedule. In addition, experienced new employees may enter somewhere midway in the scale.

Finally, do **all** employees receive regular raises or are they tied to performance standards? Good employees deserve financial recognition.

5. Do jobs with similar requirements for education, experience, hours to be worked and job stress have the same pay scales? For instance, should the dietary aid, the housekeeping aid and the nursing assistant all have the same pay schedules? Should the Director of Nursing receive more pay than the Social Worker because the size of the staff and budget is greater? In other words, on what basis have wage differentials been determined? While there are probably no precise answers to these questions, it is imperative that administrators think through these issues in order to provide a defensible rationale for decisions in these matters.

6. What benefit package is provided employees? Does it compare to

competitive organizations? Overall, benefits range from 20 percent to 40 percent of the annual salary depending on the size of the organization. Benefit packages may include paid holiday and vacation time, hospital, medical and dental insurance, retirement plans, group life insurance, educational stipends, as well as the availability of savings plans and profit sharing.

In summary, adequate wages and benefits are critical to (1) attracting competent employees to an organization, (2) keeping competent employees and (3) reducing competition from other organizations. While adequate pay scales will not substitute for other organization deficiencies, they will contribute to the hygiene of the work environment and not be a source of dissatisfaction.

SUMMARY

This chapter has been concerned with selected human resource management policies. They highlight ways to deal with common problems that both research and experience have shown to be important for healthy organizational employee relations.

REFERENCES

Chernok, Norma, "A Study of Employee Lateness." *Journal of Long-Term Care Administration,* VI:2:30–48, Summer 1978.

Herzberg, Frederick, *The Managerial Choice: To be Efficient and to be Human,* Homewood, Illinois. Dow Jones-Irwin, 1976.

Longest, B. B. and Clawson, D. E. "The Effect of Selected Factors on Hospital Turnover Rates", *Personnel Journal,* January, 1974.

Personnel Policies of Muscatine General Hospital, Muscatine, Iowa.

Snyder, Sonya M., "Controlling Absenteeism Can Help Curb Hospital Costs," *Hospitals,* Vol. 52, September 1, 1978, pp. 102–103.

Chapter 12

STAFF DEVELOPMENT

Ruth Stryker

The highest rate of turnover occurs during the first three months of employment. This is true of hospitals, nursing homes, and business organizations. Most evidence points toward two principal causes, (1) selection of the wrong person for a particular job and (2) the training and manner in which a new employee is introduced to an organization. The first reason was discussed in a previous chapter. This chapter will deal with the second cause.

The literature gives us many clues about the reasons for breakdown in employee-employer relations during the early months of employment. The endeavor to match organizational goals and values with employee goals and values is not an easy task, nor is it achieved overnight. Some researchers refer to this element as congruence or agreement of goals by both parties. This is one aspect of the process of assimilating a new person into an organization. Perhaps a more important and often overlooked aspect of job introduction relates to the socialization process. Work is not performed in a social vacuum. Therefore, far greater attention needs to be given to this basic human need on the job.

Graen and Ginsburgh introduced another way of looking at this issue. They not only examined role orientation (the tasks and work itself), but leader acceptance of the new employee also. Both were related to the assimilation process and both affected turnover.

If the greatest amount of turnover occurs during the first three months of employment, then it behooves administrators to examine organizational dynamics during this period. In other words, what in the system produces this undesired outcome? The following discussion of the practical aspects of the assimilation process is based on some of the things that are known about (1) agreement on goals and values, (2) social aspects of work, (3) job and role orientation and (4) acceptance of the new employee by the leader.

ORIENTATION

Orientation is the first step toward retention. It requires two basic aspects; one, that given to all employees and second, that part which is planned for a specific individual. For example, if you have just employed a new inexperienced nursing assistant, she will require a great deal of on-the-job training and assistance, especially during the first six weeks of employment. If at the same time, you have also employed a nursing assistant who has worked in the same capacity at another organization for five years, her training needs will obviously differ. In other words, an employee's orientation must be individually planned around the knowledge and experience he or she brings to the organization.

The quality of the initial job experience communicates a great deal about an organization. It sets the tone. It will promote displeasure with, indifference toward or regard for the organization. The outcome in terms of length of employment and job satisfaction is greatly influenced by this introduction. If negative experiences continue to dominate, leaving is an almost predictable outcome. If positive experiences predominate, the individual is likely to stay.

Orientation is comprised of several aspects. First of all, it must include an introduction to the physical environment. This means a general tour of the building so that the individual knows the general layout. The tour should emphasize obvious personal needs, such as the location of lockers, bathrooms, dining rooms, time clock, etc. It should be followed by a more in depth acquaintance with the immediate work area and with any equipment that will be used.

In addition to the physical environment, every new employee must be introduced to the people in the work environment, both employees and residents. In one's own home, you would not think of bringing in a stranger without introducing that person to anyone who lived or worked there. It is the same in a health care organization.

Orientation must also include a description of the routines with which the employee will be working. What are the meal hours for both residents and employees? What about coffee breaks? If the individual is in the housekeeping department, when is it appropriate to clean a patient's room and when should it be postponed? If the new person is a dietary worker, when are food trays prepared, delivered, collected, etc.? The new employee needs to know what the rhythm of his or her day will be.

Employees must be introduced to procedures and equipment in a planned systematic manner. If the job description is accurate, it will identify the needed content. Teaching should be spaced over a period of time so that learning occurs somewhat gradually. Too much, too soon is not only overwhelming; it is ineffective. Selected resources such as books from the library and procedure books from the station or office should be provided. Time to review them at the individual's own pace needs to be planned into the first few weeks of employment.

Every new employee should be immediately assigned to work with an experienced employee during the first week or so. This is sometimes called the buddy or hostess system. Whatever you choose to call it, it allows the new person to identify with one person as a helper. This arrangement could mean days, weeks, and sometimes months to work up to full speed or quality. The system provides someone nearby to answer questions until the job feels comfortable to the employee and until it is done well from the supervisor's viewpoint. This does not mean that two people are doing one job constantly; it means that a specific individual is designated to assist the new employee in addition to the supervisor.

The buddy system is also a way to recognize experienced employees with good work performance. Some organizations pay a slightly higher hourly rate for this recognition, while others merely use it to demonstrate confidence in the individual. The buddy must be carefully selected, as it is just as easy to learn the wrong things as the right things, and new employees will not know the difference until they are criticized for doing something wrong. Once in a while, you will find an experienced employee who finds this a burden. If so, such an assignment should not be forced, as you may lose the very employee you want to keep. In most instances, however, this responsibility is sought after when it is approached properly.

The buddy system does not absolve the supervisor or department head of responsibility to the new employee. It is simply a back up system which helps the employee to become assimilated into the work group (something that a supervisor cannot do) and to feel comfortable initially. It keeps new employees from eating alone, from feeling at loose ends, and it gives them someone to identify with until their own relationships become established.

Initial work loads should be lighter than those of experienced employees. New employees need to feel a sense of accomplishment and success. They will only have a sense of frustration and defeat if they are constantly disappointed by having to skip over things while they are learning their job and getting a feel for organizing their work.

A Negative Case in Point

This is the description of one nursing assistant's experience in a large metropolitan area nursing home of 150 beds.

I came on duty on my first day of employment at 3:00 PM. When I arrived at the nursing station, a stranger told me that I was assigned to six residents. She pointed in the direction of their rooms and walked away. No one introduced me to the staff or the residents. I then went to each resident and introduced myself because I thought that seemed like the thing to do. Throughout the evening, I had to ask each resident how to take care of them—things like which is the best side for me to stand on when you get up, where is the dining room where you eat, what time do you like to go to bed, etc. I thought it was terrible that I had to learn what to do from the residents themselves.

This nursing assistant's prior nursing home experiences had been positive, so that she was completely unprepared for this introduction to her new job. She resigned after six weeks because (1) the home did not seem to respect its residents (she never saw anyone visiting them unless they had some request or physical need), (2) the home placed the burden of orienting personnel to nursing care on the residents, (3) personnel did not help one another when there was a difficult situation, (4) there was no supervision of her work or the care and (5) there was constant bickering and tension among the staff.

I asked her what reason she gave for leaving. She told the home that her school load was heavier than anticipated, so she could not work that semester after all. If that home kept a record of leavers, they would have determined that this resignation was "employee caused," and that would have been the end of it. If that home had been aware of the need for organizational self-analysis, it would have learned something about itself. This was certainly a golden opportunity because this young woman had excellent references from her former employer and did not need them as a reference. Besides, as she put it, "I wouldn't even put that job down on my record because it would look like I had had trouble there. If another organization called them, they would have said that I had stayed only six weeks and that would not help me to locate another job." Fortunately, she had had a very positive experience at the home in which she worked in another state, so she simply found a home that was more like her prior employer.

This classic case demonstrates how recruiting, screening and selecting by itself has no relation to retention. This organization had found a good employee, but they did nothing to make the job or the organization attractive. They had ignored (1) the impact of anxiety-inducing job experiences and (2) the need for new employees to have time to assimilate knowledge and to integrate their personalities into a cohesive work group.

Parenthetically, the reader should know that the author is acquainted with the administrator of the organization involved in this story. This administrator explained in one of our classes that they did everything possible about their turnover problem. "We run ads regularly, pay bonuses, give teas and hire every ablebodied comer. Our hands are tied because all our leavers leave for personal reasons. Turnover is inevitable." As long as this tragic lack of administrative insight and refusal to analyze the internal causes of turnover persists, turnover will indeed be inevitable at this organization.

SUPERVISION OF THE NEW EMPLOYEE

The immediate supervisor or department head is responsible for a great deal of training, whether the organization has an inservice education director or not. The most convincing literature and research concludes that the basic integrity of the organization lies with the quality and quantity of communication at the supervisory level.

The supervisor must prepare a recommended outline for orientation and initial training for each position (in his or her department) in writing. It should be based on the job description and the supervisor's knowledge of what each position entails. The written plan for orientation and initial training content should be geared to the least trained and least experienced worker who might be expected to fill a particular position. It can always be modified in terms of time for the more educated and experienced new employee. This method provides each department in the organization with a written plan that details each aspect of training. Its purpose is to prevent superficial, hit or miss teaching of new employees.

The written plan should stipulate some minimum and maximum time limits. In other words, a laundry person who folds linen should not take months to learn the job, while a new administrator may need several months, not only to learn general duties but to become acquainted with the personnel, the systems, the problems and the strengths of the organization. In neither case does it mean that the worker is totally unproductive during the early weeks of employment. It merely indicates that it takes longer to learn some things than others. One can learn and do simultaneously in many instances. Nonetheless, some outside limits for teaching and learning should be specified. This will be equally helpful to the new employee.

Once the written plan for a position is developed, it can then be discussed with a new employee and specific goals can be planned for part of each day. This may range from a few minutes to a formal class. It should be most intensive during the first week or two and gradually taper off in intensity for a period of about three months. It should never just drop off, leaving the employee to dangle. Supervision is an on-going process which maintains and develops the staff of a particular department.

The supervisor needs an inservice educator to assist in carrying out initial training. Such back-up support is essential, even if the organization is small and can only afford it part time. This position should be viewed as a key resource for all supervisors and new employees. Even when such a person is available, there is nothing he or she can do about a disruptive work situation. Training cannot assist an individual to tolerate working in a department with unfair work schedules, inefficient work loads and an untrained supervisor. The training role of the supervisor will be stressed because of its critical relationship to tenure as shown by the research. Because of this emphasis, the author wishes to underscore the necessity of having an inservice educator help supervisors to plan and conduct on-the-job training. This is definitely a shared responsibility.

The following is a general guide for the first six months of employment.

First Two Weeks of Employment. This period of time might be considered a work/study period in which a new employee:

1. Receives both formal and informal instruction about the job and any equipment or procedures that are required.
2. Is assigned an hour or so for several days to read appropriate policy, equipment and procedure manuals as well as selected articles or books related to the job.
3. Is assigned to work with another employee (the hostess employee or buddy).
4. Is assigned to independent regularly scheduled work but with a somewhat reduced work load. This can be increased gradually on the basis of a decision made jointly by the employee, the supervisor, the inservice person, and perhaps the buddy.

5. Meets with the supervisor at the end of each week to determine the needs and progress of the individual.

WEEKS THREE THROUGH SIX. Weekly conferences with the supervisor should continue. These conferences need not be lengthy, but they should not be done on the run or in passing. The purpose of continued conferences is to identify any further learning goals, feeling of confidence, any interpersonal problems encountered, and general adjustment. They should be discussed from the point of view of both the employee and the supervisor. The supervisor's role is to support the individual, not to undermine with judgmental observations or evaluations. This can be accomplished by conveying acceptance and a desire to coach and assist in any weak areas. It also provides an opportunity to give positive comments about the quality of work done.

Early problems can be approached as goals to be achieved in the upcoming week. When conferences are regularly scheduled, the impulse to call someone in only when there is a problem is averted. There is a long-run effect of early and planned conferences; they set in motion a supervisor/subordinate relationship based on mutual interest in the person, and an interest in good work as well as poor work. This lays the ground work for better communications in the future. If the supervisor is approachable early on, the employee will feel freer to discuss problems at a later date. If adequate help is given initially and a good relationship has been launched, the employee is more likely to bring up future problems rather than let them smoulder.

WEEKS SEVEN THROUGH TWELVE. Supervisor conferences begin to taper off to two, three and then four week intervals. The general tone and purpose are the same as in previous weeks.

WEEKS THIRTEEN THROUGH TWENTY-SIX. These are crucial weeks, as the employee is, for the most part, left on his own. During this time, the individual comes to terms with the work group. It is now that the employee chooses friends, decides to become an informal group leader or not, notices if the supervisor has favorites and integrates his or her personal life with work. During this period, the employee decides whether there is congruence or agreement about job expectations and what the job actually offers. This is true across all job levels. For instance, if a professional person expects to use higher levels of skill than the job allows, he or she may request greater responsibility.

It is also at this time that an individual can become bored. The challenge of learning is pretty much over and the overly qualified person becomes restless. Managers should realize that a poor matching of an individual's intellectual ability and ambition with the job will show up at this time. If there was a good match, the person is likely to stay. If not, the person will be looking for a new challenge and will be interested in leaving or being promoted. If the job holds little or no opportunity for promotion, the less ambitious person is probably the best choice if turnover during the third to sixth months is high. This, of course, assumes that all of the factors discussed thus far have been considered.

INSERVICE EDUCATION

During the first months of employment, the role of the inservice educator includes helping to plan orientation schedules, conducting facility tours, teaching formal classes and locating resources for the various departments. Because so many inservice positions are filled by nurses, there is a tendency to neglect the needs of other departments. However, classes on body mechanics, safety, fire and disaster procedures, confidentiality, and many other topics are needed by all employees. The job description and budget for this position should not be limited to the nursing department in any health care organization.

The inservice educator must have had or obtained some teacher training. If not, he or she will have very limited vision and skill on the job. Courses in teaching adults and leading group discussions are not difficult to locate, nor are they expensive. Nearly all area vocational schools, community colleges and state colleges and universities offer such courses. Some professional associations and the Red Cross also offer courses in some localities.

Whether the inservice department has several staff; one person full time (or part time) or shares staff with a hospital or another nursing home, such a department is essential. Not only must the educator understand how adults learn and possess some teaching skills, this person must also have knowledge of the needs of the special clientele being served.

In the case of the nursing home, knowledge about the well elderly, the physically disabled elderly, the mentally impaired elderly, and rehabilitative and environmental measures must be in hand. An educator cannot be expected to be all-knowing about everything. Therefore, the primary task is to know resources. These can be in the form of books, journals, audiovisual materials, persons in the community or employees within the organization.

The actual role of the educator has many facets. Some of the primary responsibilities include:

1. Assisting with work-related problem solving.
2. Improving on-the-job skill and performance.
3. Developing all staff to grow with organizational changes.
4. Helping staff to understand and handle their emotional reactions to feelings of inadequacy, hopelessness, anger and grief.
5. Helping staff to accept the attitudes and feelings of others by not inflicting their values on others and yet maintain their own values. (This problem becomes especially apparent when residents are sexually active.)
6. Gathering resources for the training needs of all staff, which of course includes the needs of department heads untrained in management.
7. Orienting and participating in the teaching of all new personnel on all shifts. This implies flexible hours for this person.
8. Assist in career development and promotion of individuals who need greater personal and professional goals.

Inservice educator time is often consumed by training nursing assistants in nursing homes. This is most unfortunate as it limits the scope of the job not only to one department but to one position. In addition, repetitious teaching combined with high turnover is unrewarding. There is simply no time or energy to go beyond the basics so residents lose out and organizational performance remains at a standstill.

Many states either offer courses or require training of geriatric nursing assistants. Because many of these curricula are minimal, some nursing homes either prefer to teach their own programs or elect to build upon them. If administrative procedures for hiring practices are well planned, nursing assistant programs can be set on a regular schedule to minimize the repetition of this task. Some homes jointly sponsor such programs in order to free up time for the inservice educator to attend to other responsibilities.

PERFORMANCE APPRAISAL

The purpose of performance appraisal is to improve the job performance of employees. It is a part of staff development, but is seldom thought of as such. However, personnel experts agree that many systems fall short of this goal, mainly because they so often place the supervisor in the untenable position of judging the worth of subordinates. This aspect of conventional appraisal programs produces widespread uneasiness on the part of both the employee to be evaluated and the person doing the evaluation.

A sounder approach must be adopted, one which places responsibility on the subordinate for establishing performance goals and appraising progress toward them. In addition to avoiding the major weaknesses mentioned above, appraising must also take other factors into consideration if the organization is to stimulate the development of the employee.

The attainment of optimum performance by an employee involves factors within that individual AND those in the organization. While an individual's ability affects performance, there is little he or she can do about that; other factors are within the person's control, however. By the same token, the job structure and organizational relationships are within the control of the organization. Therefore, a manager who appraises an employee must appraise all of the factors, including his or her influence in relation to an individual employee's performance on the job.

In general, there is no known panacea for performance appraisal. However, most systems can be improved by addressing three of the most commonly found problems:

1. There should be frequent feedback, not just in the form of an annual evaluation. Any feedback that tends to discourage, alienate or patronize should be avoided.
2. Keep the approach to evaluation future-oriented rather than rehashing the past. Positive suggestions from both the supervisor and the subordinate for future goals and ways of accomplishing them should be emphasized. Remember, the vast majority of employees want to perform at their highest capacity and they want to perform well.
3. The appraisal form itself should not contain trait oriented items that require subjective judgments that tend to insult rather than instruct. The form should contain observable objective and measurable performance standards TAKEN FROM THE JOB DESCRIPTION.

A recommended approach to performance appraisal is that of the Work Plan & Review (WPR). There are variations on implementation, but the major thrust is to make it a joint planning session with the involvement of both the supervisor and subordinate. In order to accomplish this, five steps are recommended.

Step 1—Together, both should review the job description to make sure that there is agreement on the major areas of responsibility and accountability. Step 2—The employee sets performance targets for the next few months or year. Step 3—The employee again meets with the supervisor to discuss these targets and they select ways of measuring progress. Step 4—checkpoints for measuring progress are established. Step 5—they meet at the end of the period to discuss the results of the targeted goals. The process can then be repeated.

Properly executed, performance appraisals can become a useful management tool. While the major purpose is employee development, they can also help to identify persons for promotion, demotion, transfer and executive development. They can be used by the training director to identify training needs, and finally, they can help to identify persons for merit raises, special bonuses and special recognition.

SUMMARY

Once the organization has recruited, screened, and selected the best, or perhaps the most appropriate person for a particular position, it is incumbent on the inservice educator and the supervisor to plan and provide the best possible work environment for learning. While this should involve the input of an inservice educator, the primary focus should be on the application of learning to the job. Close supervision during the early weeks and months of employment are crucial if the organization wishes to retain its employees during the highest turnover period, the first three months. These measures, along with on-going inservice education, will reduce the amount of job stress and anxiety and tend to increase both the tenure and organizational committment of employees. Finally, a good performance appraisal system will help to develop individual employees to their fullest capacity. The ultimate goal ofcourse is to enable the organization to provide high quality care to residents.

REFERENCES

Burke, Robert E. et al. "Research Brief: Training Geriatric Nursing Assistants— A Solution," *Journal of Long-Term Care Administration,* VIII:3:37–41, Fall 1980.

Graen, George and Ginsburgh, Steven, "Job Resignation as a Function of Role Orientation and Leader Acceptance: A Longitudinal Investigation of Organizational Acceptance," *Organizational Behavior and Human Performance,* 19:1–17, 1977.

Kellogg, Marion. *Closing the Performance Gap.* American Management Association, New York, 1967.

Performance Appraisal. Harvard Business Review, a special issue, a classic, 1972.

Porter, L.W. et al., "Organizational Commitment and Managerial Turnover: A Longitudianl Study," *Organizational Behavior and Human Performance,* 15:87–98, 1976.

RECOMMENDED RESOURCES

Books

Ernst, Nora and Helen West. *Nursing Home Staff Development, A Guide for Inservice Programs.* New York, Springer Publishing Co., 1983.

Food Service Worker and *Housekeeping Aide.* Hospital Research and Educational Trust, 840 North Lake Shore Drive, Chicago, Illinois 60611. A student manual and an instructor's guide is available for each. One book is for the food service worker and one is for the housekeeping aide. Each describes techniques of the job and basic considerations for performance.

Lobsenz, N.M. *Sex After Sixty-Five.* Public Affairs Pamphlet No. 519, Public Affairs Pamphlets, 381 Park Avenue South, New York, NY 10016, 1975.

Training and Continuing Education: A Handbook for Health Care Institutions. Hospital and Research Educational Trust, 840 North Lake Shore Drive, Chicago, Illinois, 60611. A text for staff education directors, discusses the teaching and learning process, methods of teaching, writing objectives, evaluation methods, etc.

Journals

Concern
Generations
Gerontologist
Geriatric Nursing
Journal of Gerontological Nursing
Journal of Long-Term Care Administration
Modern Health Care
The Provider

Chapter 13

MONITORING AND EVALUATING HR PRACTICES

Ruth Stryker

THE CLIMATE OF LONG–TERM CARE
AS A WORK ENVIRONMENT

Every employer must be cognizant of inherent factors that influence employees in a particular work environment. First, one must acknowledge the negative factors. For example, nursing home work is not easy work emotionally or physically, yet it is both challenging and satisfying to many workers. Pressure by external agencies often forces nursing homes to fill vacancies quickly and thus encourages the hiring of inappropriate or younger workers who are known to turn over rapidly in any organization.

Nursing homes have gone through rapid change during the past decade. They have become heavily regulated yet some regulations, such as staffing ratios, have not changed much in spite of the fact that resident populations are sicker, more debilitated and over ten years older than they were a decade ago. Nursing homes have been encouraged to provide higher quality care but with a preponderance of unskilled workers.

All of this seems to suggest that nursing home administrators have some very special tasks. They obviously need to develop competitive pay scales, fringe benefits, equitable distribution of less popular work times etc. However, the need to control public spending conflicts with some of these goals as well as some of the standards set by law.

Public image also influences nursing homes. The poor practices of some have been widely described in the media. This has an impact on the self-esteem of persons who work in nursing homes. The average citizen is ill-equipped to judge whether a home is good or bad. Non-professional employees are poorly trained and often unaware of facts about the aged and their diseases. Unfortunately, some professional

154

health workers carry similar misconceptions about geriatric care because of the dearth of professional expertise in this field.

The high proportion of non-professional workers to professional workers in nursing homes results in the fact that most direct care is given by non-professional workers. This creates a circularity of nursing home problems. A small number of supervisors must do more supervision, especially in the nursing department, and opportunities to learn better supervisory skills are also inadequate.

Finally, patient outcomes are not likely to be dramatic, and death can be anticipated for many. However, the goal of rehabilitation or at least improved function must be coupled with helping to provide meaning to the lives of residents, maintaining comfort, and enhancing self esteem and dignity.

There are other factors that make the climate of geriatric work unique, but the above mentioned must be continually addressed by the administrator and department heads. Remember, these obstacles are shared by all homes. Quality homes with good personnel relations and low turnover experience the same external problems as poor nursing homes with high turnover. Therefore, it is the immediate work environment that must be scrutinized.

The work environment in geriatric organizations not only affects employees but it also influences the welfare of residents directly. Therefore, governing boards, administrators, owners and department heads must be willing to analyze their own organizations, monitor their own practices and take appropriate actions in order to develop new organizational strengths. Those who are willing to do this will find cost benefits, improved quality of resident care and a richer work environment for their employees and for themselves. One of several ways to diagnose a host of human resource management problems is to investigate turnover and related indicators in depth. This method will be the approach in this chapter.

HOW MUCH TURNOVER IS ACTUALLY AVOIDABLE?

Unless your turnover is under 20 or 25 percent, you undoubtedly have avoidable turnover. Because of the greater proportion of non-professional employees, nursing homes will usually have a somewhat higher turnover rate than hospitals because professional employees tend to have lower turnover rates in almost all occupations. Therefore, 20 or 25 percent would be considered high hospital turnover.

HIGH turnover is organizationally caused in spite of reasons employees give for leaving. Therefore, rather than excusing it, administrators and department heads must identify the causes and attend to them appropriately.

After studying turnover, Asis concluded that 65 percent of all turnover is avoidable. Peskin says that unavoidable turnover, that is, turnover caused by transfers, relocation, change in marital status, etc. accounts for a small fraction of turnover. Fournet, another researcher, uses the terms "voluntary" and "involuntary" (personal and not job-related causes of leaving). When this author studied reasons for leaving in twenty-five nursing homes, only about one quarter of the separations were for reasons that could be classified as involuntary (unavoidable). This meant that for these homes, 75 percent of their separations were voluntary (avoidable). All of these studies have remarkably similar findings; namely, at least two-thirds of all turnover is voluntary and avoidable.

In your home, why do personnel leave? It is imperative that you try to find out. Whether you inquire through exit interviews by someone removed from the immediate work situation or by an anonymous followup letter, it is crucial information that can help you to select some of your administrative interventions. Remember, many employees will be reluctant to give their real reasons for leaving if they fear a poor recommendation. However, if you continue to ask enough leavers, you will find some real reasons and you may even find some consistency.

Usually you will find that the voluntary or avoidable separation does not leave for one but for several reasons. Reflect back on some job that you left. It is quite likely the factors in the situation "piled up" before you made the decision to resign. Your employees are no different. For instance, a dietary aide may first find that she had to learn the job the "hard way"; then find that the supervisor has favorites when it comes to assigning undesirable hours; discovers that there is so much bickering among staff that she tries to stay aloof from the others; and finally decides to quit when the supervisor bawls her out in front of the cook for something that she had never been told about; in addition, the pay was low. When such a person is asked to give the reason for leaving, he or she may say "to seek a better job", to "earn more money" or any number of other fairly acceptable reasons. A well conducted exit interview will attempt to find out as many reasons for leaving as possible in order to have as many facts as possible.

Exit interviews may not be necessary for every departing employee. For instance, if the dietary department has a high turnover rate regularly each quarter, problems obviously exist. When this occurs, you can interview at least one departing employee in depth and with honesty and candor. You might say, "I am concerned about the high turnover in our dietary department. There are obviously some problems that I should know more about in order to deal with them better." You may want to state that you want to improve the situation so that the organization does not lose persons with his or her qualities. This approach is likely to produce a fairly honest response, as the employee will be less fearful of a poor letter of reference.

In summary, the majority of terminations from organizations with annual turnover over 20 percent are due to avoidable causes. They usually leave for multiple reasons, not just one. It is to the interest of the administrator to find out why personnel leave that organization. All information should be recorded and then shared with each department head.

CALCULATING INDICATORS

The first step is to look at the organization as a whole and then at each department. Monitoring absenteeism, turnover, wastage and stability of personnel is a management information tool. It can be used to diagnose certain organizational ailments. It needs to be done quarterly, not just occasionally. It must be done by department and/or unit and shift, not just for the entire organization.

What can be learned from this management data? First of all, you can identify trouble spots. If most of your problems are in one department, one section of a department, on a particular shift or among one classification of employees, you know where to start. If you have had low turnover, you know when there is a change. By sharing this information with other homes and hospitals, you know how you compare with other organizations. The administrator must share this information with department heads, obtain their observations and make sure they know their responsibility in the matter. Then management can begin to work together.

First, how do you calculate these indicators? The following are commonly used formulas.

Turnover Rate:

$$\frac{\text{no. of leavers during the quarter}}{\text{*average no. on payroll for quarter}} \times 100 \text{ rate for quarter}$$

Example:

$$\frac{\text{no. of leavers 10/1 through 12/31} = 40}{200\,(10/1) + 196\,(11/1) + 198\,(12/1) = 594 \div 3 = 198\,(\text{av. no. on payroll 10/1--12/31})}$$

$$\frac{40}{198} \quad .202 \times 100 = 20.2\% \text{ T.O. rate 10/1--12/31}$$

If you wish to estimate your annual turnover rate, multiply the quarterly rate by 4. In this case, the estimated annual T.O. would be 80.8 percent.

The reason for calculating T.O. quarterly is to find out if you have recurring seasonal changes, to evaluate any organizational changes and to help long-range staffing plans.

There are many ways of computing turnover rates. The above formula can be used when the number of employees vary only slightly during the months that are being measured. However, for large organizations with wider fluctuations of numbers of employees, the following formula is more commonly used:

$$\text{T.O.} = \frac{c}{\dfrac{a + b}{2}}$$

In this formula:

    a = no. on payroll at the beginning of the time period being measured
    b = no. on payroll at the end of the time period being measured
    c = no. of separations during the time period being measured

Example:

$$\frac{125\,(\text{separations})}{\dfrac{650\,(1/1) + 600\,(3/31)}{2}} = \frac{125}{\dfrac{1250}{2}} = \frac{125}{625} = .20 \times 100 = 20\%$$

Stability Rate:

$$\frac{\text{no. of persons (from below) who have been there 12 mo.}}{\text{total no. on payroll on last day of quarter}} \times 100 = \text{S.R.}$$

Example:

$$\frac{60\,(\text{on payroll since 12/31/88})}{100\ \text{on payroll on 12/31/89}} = 60 \div 100 = .60 \times 100 = 60\% \text{ S.R.}$$

---

*Calculate by adding the number on the payroll at the beginning (or end, but be consistent) of each month in the quarter and divide by 3.

Note: Your stability rate is always an annual calculation. By monitoring it quarterly, you can see whether it fluctuates with your T.O. rate and see to what extent your organizational inputs change your S.R. Remember, your stability rate actually reflects what you did six to twelve months ago.

Wastage Rate: concentrates on new employees only. Because our research in long-term care administration suggests that most employees leave during the first three to six months of employment, it can be useful. It is calculated as follows:

$$\frac{\text{no. of newly hired who leave}}{\text{no. of newly hired}} \times 100 = \text{W.R.}$$

Absentee Rate:

Absenteeism, a less than final withdrawal from an organization, is also very costly. The cost of overtime or replacement personnel, the decline in employee morale, work disruption and decreased productivity waste time and dollars. In many instances, it also reduces the quality of care. Every organization should monitor its absenteeism rate. This is calculated by using a formula similar to the turnover and stability rate formulae. It is as follows:

$$\frac{\text{Number of days absent}}{\text{Number of days worked}} \times 100$$

It is recommended that only the first five days of an extended absence be counted in order to prevent the figure from overrepresenting one or two persons with a lengthy illness. Most organizations attempt to approach an absence rate of around 2 percent.

In addition to keeping track of the absence rate of the organization, the frequency of absences by individuals should be examined by supervisors. Obviously one ten-day absence is very different from ten one-day absences. Supervisors should not only keep a record of absences and the reasons, but look for individual patterns (before or after a day off, after payday, on the same weekday, etc.). Individuals with such a pattern should be counseled and it should be made clear that it is disruptive to the work situation and will not be tolerated if it continues.

Figure 13-1 shows a quarterly record form that can be kept by the person who maintains your personnel records. It should be noted that if you calculate T.O. quarterly, you sum the four quarters to obtain the annual rate. For example:

DEPARTMENT	TERMINATIONS			AVERAGE NO. EMPLOYEES			TURNOVER RATE		
	Part-time	Full-time	Total	Part-time	Full-time	Total	Part-time	Full-time	Total
Nursing									
Unit A									
Unit B									
Unit C									
Dietary									
Housekeeping									
Laundry									
Activities									
Office									
Maintenance									
Others									
Total Org.									
Nursing by									
Days									
Evenings									
Nights									
Reasons									
Worker caused									
Competition									
Job caused									
Discharges									

Figure 13-1. Quarterly turnover record for the period

January 1 through March 31	12%
April 1 through June 30	17%
July 1 through September 30	20%
October 1 through December 31	15%
This year's T.O. rate	= 64%

WHAT CAN YOU LEARN FROM YOUR DATA?

Once you have obtained your information, what assumptions can you make from it? Because every organization has individual problems, let us look at the quarterly summary of two organizations.

Organization A

Department Separations

<u>10</u> Nursing
<u>7</u> Dietary
<u>4</u> Housekeeping
<u>3</u> Activities
<u>6</u>
<u>30</u> Total

T.O. Rate

17% (Nursing)
35% (Dietary)
50% (Housekeeping)
100% (activities)
All others
30% (120% estimate annually) based on average no. of employees = 100

Age of leavers

<u>24</u> 24 or under
<u>3</u> 25–44
<u>1</u> 45–64
<u>2</u> 65 or over

Length of stay

<u>21</u> 3 mo. or less
<u>6</u> 4–11 months
<u>1</u> 1–3 years
<u>2</u> 3 or more years

Stability rate — 45%
Wastage rate — 58%
Absenteeism — 5%

Causes

<u>4</u> Worker cause
<u>7</u> Competition
<u>8</u> Job caused
<u>8</u> Discharges
<u>4</u> Worker cause
<u>7</u> Competition
<u>8</u> Job caused
<u>8</u> Discharges

What does this report tell you about Organization A? It tells a great deal, indeed. Here are a few highlights that can help you to read your own summary sheets.

NAME	Job title	Department	Age	Marital status	Shift worked	Years	Months	Moved	Married	Needed at home	Ill	Injured	Retired	Seek better job	Attend school	Transportation difficult	
EMPLOYEE DATA						**TENURE**		**WORKER CAUSED**									
								Family			Health			Competition			

Figure 13-2. Worksheet

JOB CAUSED														DISCHARGES			OTHER	
Wage & Hours				The Job									Supv.	Con-duct	Perfor-mance			
Rate of pay	Too much overtime	Poor work environment	Unsettled grievance	Change in org.	Work too hard	Too much to learn	Too much responsibility	No security	No future	Work depressing	Work unsatisfying	Dislike supervisor	Dislike employees	Inappropriate behavior	Excessive absenteeism	Unable to learn	Poor quality work	

Figure 13-2 *(continued)*

CATEGORY	81 (Q1)	81 (Q2)	81 (Q3)	81 (Q4)	82 (Q1)	82 (Q2)	82 (Q3)	82 (Q4)
DEPARTMENTAL QUITS								
Nursing								
Dietary								
Housekeeping								
P.T.								
Social Service								
Activities								
Maintenance								
Laundry								
Clerical								
Other								
TOTAL								
AGE								
25 or under								
26 - 45								
46 - 64								
65 or over								
LENGTH OF STAY								
3 mos. or less								
4 - 12 months								
13 - 35 months								
3 years or more								
NURS. JOB TITLE								
R.N.								
L.P.N.								
Nurs. Asst.								
CAUSES								
Worker Caused								
Competition								
Attend School								
Job Caused								
Discharged								
TURNOVER BY DEPT.								
Nursing								
Dietary								
Housekeeping								
QUARTER'S T.O.								
QUARTER'S S.R.								

Figure 13-3. Administrator's cumulative record of turnover.

1. With a stability rate of 45 percent (only 45% of the staff having been there for a year or more) and a T.O. rate of 120 percent, a wastage rate of 58% and 5 percent absenteeism, you have certain jobs turning over not once or twice but three or four times a year in some instances.

2. This seems to be happening in the dietary, housekeeping and activities departments. Note, while nursing has more separations, it has the lowest T.O. rate. You are therefore sure that your wastage rate also relates to the other three departments. What causes the high turnover in these three departments? Inadequate leadership by the department head? Informal group pressure on new employees? Inadequate standards, supervision and training? Poor selection? In other words, this tells you **where** to look for problems and suggests certain possibilities that the administrator and department head must discuss.

3. The many young leavers suggests that it might be worthwhile to try to attract more older workers.

4. Most leavers staying less than three months suggests rather immediate dissatisfaction and that either lack of supervision and/or training are causing some of the problems.

5. That about one third left because of the job suggests that you should talk to leavers to find out what job factors caused them to leave. Another one third being discharged suggests that screening and selection factors are inadequate.

Organization B

Department Separations
20 Nursing
_1 Dietary
10 Housekeeping
31 Total

T.O. Rate
20%
5%
80%
20% (80% estimate annually) based on average no. of employees = 155

Age of leavers
14 24 or under
14 25–44
_3 45–64
_0 65 or over

Length of stay
14 3 months or less
14 4–11 months
_3 1–3 years
_0 3 or more years

Causes
_6 worker caused
_7 competition
16 job caused
_1 discharges

Stability rate—85%
Wastage rate—14%
Absentee rate—2%

Organization B has a very different set of problems even though the number of separations is almost identical.

1. With a stability rate of 85 percent, why is the turnover rate 80 percent? This means that all of the turnover is accounted for in 15 percent of the jobs. This means that turnover can be reduced by looking at a small segment of the organization, in this case, housekeeping and nursing.
2. The age of leavers is fairly well distributed so that does not seem to be a selection factor.
3. The length of stay of leavers shows rather immediate dissatisfaction and there is a high number of job-related reasons for leaving. Since the administrator must look at only two departments, housekeeping in particular, it should not be difficult to find out what is wrong.

Neither of these organizations is ficticious. Therefore, the administrator findings can be described along with the actual outcomes. In the case of Organization A, the administrator found many problems and it took a year before he was able to reverse the indicators. Actually, he found a department head who was unwilling to discipline a trouble-making employee in the housekeeping department. He provided supervisory training for the department head who learned how to contain this individual. In the dietary department, he found no planned or itemized program for training new employees. He and the inservice director worked with the department head to prepare a planned orientation and training checklist for the department. The administrator was in charge of the activities department, a job that he obviously was neglecting because of time commitments. He developed one individual on the staff to direct the program, thus relieving himself of doing a task he was doing poorly.

Organization B had a much simpler task, but it was not a pleasant one. After working with the housekeeping supervisor for several months, the administrator finally asked for her resignation. This person should never have been promoted to the position and was found incapable of directing the work of others in spite of the help given. The major nursing department problem was located on the evening shift of one unit. It had to do with staff problems with two distressed families who complained regularly and disturbed the resident on many occasions. The social worker and director of nursing found ways to help the families and to assist the staff to deal with the families. The staff learned ways of handling both the families and their own behavior. This of course reduced the problem as well as gave the staff a sense of growth and new confidence.

These two organizational cases demonstrate 1) how individualized employee problems can be, 2) what a broad range of skills administrators and department heads must have, 3) that key indicators provide HR information that help to locate internal problems, and 4) the data itself almost identifies what the administrative actions should be.

SUMMARY

The basic components of HRM are usually considered to be 1) recruitiment, screening and selection of employees, 2) job descriptions, 3) personnel policies, 4) performance appraisal, 5) compensation systems, 6) employee relations, and 7) organizational development. There are many indicators of success or lack of success in these areas. This chapter has dealt with only three; properly used, however, they can help the administrator to locate weaknesses and strengths in nearly all of the major areas that are considered a part of human resource management.

REFERENCES

Asis, L.B., "A Study of Employee Turnover" as quoted in Basil S. Georgopoulos, *Hospital Organization Research; Review and Source Book*, Philadelphia, PA, Saunders, 1975, pp 305–306.

Fournet, G. P. et al.: Job Satisfaction: Issues and Problems," *Personnel Psychology*, 19:2:165, 1966.

Halbur, Bernice and Neil Fears. "Nursing Personnel Turned Over: Potential Positive Effects on Resident Outcomes in Nursing Homes," *Gerontologist* 26:1, February, 1986.

Hall, Douglas T. and James G. Goodale. *Human Resource Management*, Glenview, IL, Scott, Foresman, 1985.

Peskin, D. *Doomsday Job — The Behavioral Anatomy of Turnover*, American Management Association, 1973.

PART IV

CREATING THE ENVIRONMENT FOR HEALTH CARE

In aggregate, geriatric residents require services from a host of health care professions. Physical therapy, occupational therapy, recreational therapy, audiology, speech therapy, psychology, psychiatry, dentistry, podiatry, dietetics, pharmacy, the clergy and others are usually provided by part-time personnel or consultants except in larger organizations. Rather than attempt to deal with such a multitude of services, only four have been selected for examination. They are medical care, nursing care, social services, and activities (chapters 14, 15, 16, and 17).

In addition, physical and psychosocial function are strongly influenced by the physical environment. Chapter 18, Environmental Adaptations to Compensate for Sensory Changes, discusses ways in which more supportive or prosthetic surroundings can improve function.

Geriatric health care is viewed by these authors as a complex interaction between professional care givers, the physical environment, and the physical and mental function of its residents. Administrative initiative can influence all of these factors.

Chapter 14

MEDICAL CARE AND THE
ROLE OF THE MEDICAL DIRECTOR

Ruth Stryker

MEDICAL CARE ISSUES

There are two major impediments to medical care of the aged; 1) the education and interest of the attending physician, and 2) the beliefs of elderly clients regarding their symptoms. Earlier chapters discussed several studies of physician interest and knowledge of aging. Lack of interest and stereotyping the aged were in part due to lack of exposure to geriatric content in school. To alter this situation, medical schools are rapidly beginning to include geriatric medicine in their curricula. However, in 1982 only about one-third (45) of the nation's medical schools offered electives in geriatric medicine. Moreover, only 2.5 percent of America's 16,000 medical students took one of these elective courses.

In an initiative in 1987 to alter this situation, the American Board of Internal Medicine and the American Board of Family Practice formed an alliance to begin a standard for the certification of their diplomates in geriatric medicine. Beginning in 1988, examinations to qualify for a Certificate of Added Qualifications in geriatrics became available. For the first five years, diplomates from these Boards having a substantial geriatric practice may sit for the examination. After that time, physicians will be required to have an additional two-year geriatric residency to be eligible for the examination.

Currently, there are just a handful of fully qualified geriatricians in the United States, and most of them are medical school faculty. This of course means that the vast majority of practicing physicians have never had a formal course in geriatric medicine although many have sought out continuing education programs to compensate for deficits in their basic medical education. Many family practitioners and internists attending the elderly have both an interest in the aged and a commitment to further their knowledge of the field. Administrators of geriatric health services must of course screen their physicians, especially their medical directors, for both of these qualities.

The second issue regarding medical care relates to the elderly patient and the way diseases are manifested in the aged. For example, many older persons take pain for granted. They know that stiff and aching joints are common, so they attribute physical symptoms to being old and therefore, do not seek medical help. On the other hand, certain conditions present either no symptoms or symptoms that differ from those in younger age groups. A silent heart attack is an example.

It is often very difficult to distinguish manifestations of the aging process from a disease when it occurs in the altered physiology of an older person. Even a physician must be on guard for errors. When the 85-year old square dancer's doctor said his painful right knee was due to aging, the old man retorted that his left knee was just as old. Whether this story is true or not, it serves to remind us all that aging is not a disease.

An older person's physiological response to either a prescription or over-the-counter drug is not always known or predictable, as drug testing is done on young adults. Also, older persons usually see more than one doctor so they may end up taking multiple prescriptions in addition to self-prescribed over-the-counter drugs. In combination, this is often detrimental and may even result in contradictory reactions in the body. When these things occur, a patient is likely to stop taking a drug because of an unpleasant reaction or because "it doesn't do any good."

Older persons frequently require smaller dosages of medication than those usually recommended for adults. The absorption, distribution, metabolism and excretion of drugs change with age. This is one of the reasons for requiring a pharmacist to review medication use in long term care facilities.

It is critical that health care professionals identify ALL the drugs a patient takes. To accomplish this, many physicians request that all drugs be brought to the office in a plastic bag. Thus, the physician can check for outdated drugs and possible drug-drug interactions. This also provides an opportunity to discuss the purpose of a regimen and to monitor its success and compliance. These issues are critical to the care of elderly persons in all types of residential settings, including the home.

COMMON MEDICAL PROBLEMS OF THE ELDERLY

PHYSICAL PROBLEMS

The interaction of acute and chronic illnesses and the psychosocial components of disability create a medical challenge for all health care professionals dealing with the elderly. Common geriatric medical diagnoses are arthritis, cardiovascular problems, diabetes, fractures, stroke, perceptual deficits and infections of the upper respiratory and urinary tracts. These conditions require diagnostic lab and x-ray procedures, surgery if indicated, and appropriate medical treatment. While much of this sounds like traditional medical care, there are many differences. In addition to the cautions cited in previous paragraphs, elderly persons have multiple diagnoses (a principal reason for the high incidence of polypharmacy) their symptoms often differ or are absent, and their laboratory results may differ from standardized norms.

Ronald Cape, a geriatrician, classifies geriatric conditions by the most frequent problems occurring in the aged; 1) falls, 2) iatrogenic conditions (those caused by the care or treatment of a condition), 3) confusion, 4) incontinence, and 5) homeostatic impairments. He proposes that physicians work toward a diagnosis from a better knowledge of the causes of these manifestations.

In addition to a medical diagnosis and treatment plan, a functional assessment is necessary to determine what a person can do in terms of ADL's (dressing, bathing, eating, grooming, toileting), ambulation, and Instrumental Activities of Living (IADL's) such as general care of the environment, shopping, food preparation, and the ability to do personal finances. From these assessments, one can 1) identify environmental changes that will increase functional abilities, 2) suggest areas of rehabilitation, and 3) recommend the appropriate type of residential setting.

MENTAL/EMOTIONAL PROBLEMS

A review of medical records in any nursing home will produce a varied list of diagnoses including senile dementia, chronic/organic brain syndrome, cerebroarteriosclerotic brain disease, and Alzheimer's disease. The behaviors which elicit such diagnoses are usually described as confusion, disorientation, wandering, incoherent speech, poor judgment, sloppiness, inattentiveness, being physically and/or verbally abusive, etc. However, the mere presence of such symptoms do not justify such diagnoses without additional information and evidence.

It is necessary to determine the underlying causes of behaviors, seek a correct diagnosis and identify treatment and management measures. Diagnostic errors can cause further limitations and deprive patients from successful treatment outcomes. There are three major classifications of problems in this area: dementia, delirium, and depression. The management and care of these conditions are all very different, yet symptoms can be remarkably similar.

Dementia: Dementia is a syndrome that features chronic, generalized, deterioration of previously acquired intellectual activities and interferes with social and/or occupational functioning due to changes in the brain. Impairment of memory, abstract thinking, and judgment is evident in a fully developed case, as is defective impulse control and either accentuation or alteration of previous personality traits.

The symptoms appear so gradually that patients and families find it almost impossible to specify the time of onset. At first, symptoms are merely baffling so help is not sought until the patient does not recognize a friend or is unable to manage the checkbook. The clinical course may be progressive, static, or partly or fully remitting and can last up to 20 years. The incidence increases with age and now constitutes the fourth leading cause of death in the United States.

There are several causes of dementias. Alzheimer's Type accounts for 50 to 60 percent of all cases. Its cause is unknown. The irreversible and progressive neuropathologic changes in the brain correlate with the decreasing abilities of the patient. The immediate cause of death is usually a respiratory infection. Because an accurate diagnosis can only be made by autopsy, the diagnosis is made by excluding other conditions. Family members should be encouraged to consider authorizing an autopsy as it is one way to learn more about these conditions, identify family incidence, and evaluate the accuracy of diagnostic measures.

Multi-infarct dememtias caused by infarctions and small thrombi that damage or destroy brain cells with resulting damage to mental function account for another 20 percent of these conditions. It is important to diagnose and treat any problem such as hypertension which could lead to the infarcts. The aim is to try to stop continued progress of the condition, but there is no way to reverse damage that has already occurred.

Less frequent causes of dementia include Subdural Hematoma (possibly resulting from a fall), Dementia Pugilistica (from repeated head trauma as seen in some boxers), neurosyphilis, and other conditions. Some of these conditions are reversible which is the reason for identifying the cause before irreversible brain damage occurs.

Delirium: Delirium can occur at any age and is characterized by rapid onset of disturbances of attention, memory, thinking, perception, orientation, psychomotor activity, and the sleep-wakefulness cycle. This syndrome has also been known as acute organic brain syndrome. There are fluctuating periods of lethargy and hyperactivity, and the patient may appear quite lucid at intervals.

Major causes include drug toxicity (often from psychotropic drugs, digitalis, diuretics, anti-hypertensives and others), central nervous system diseases, cardiopulmonary diseases, anemia, "silent" heart attack, diabetes, infections, postoperative state, or fecal impaction. In addition to the more clearly designated clinical causes of delirium, there are psychosocial causes, e.g. situations which cause over- or under-stimulation, such as being cared for in an intensive care unit or convalescing in a darkened, quiet room.

Once the cause is identified, the underlying condition can be treated. This reversible disorder rarely lasts more than one month.

Depression: Depression is evidenced by a dejected mood, psychomotor retardation, insomnia, weight loss, feelings of guilt, and somatic preoccupations with constipation, fatigue and insomnia. Depression is the major psychiatric disturbance in the elderly. Unfortunately, it is sometimes confused with dementia or, it is sometimes thought to be somatic and may be treated with a laxative. When it is properly diagnosed, depressed elderly respond to treatment very well. This is even true when depression and dementia co-exist.

EVALUATION, DIAGNOSIS, AND TREATMENT

Evaluation and Diagnosis: It is essential that a careful diagnostic work-up be done for each patient prior to diagnosis. It is also important to keep in mind that a person with dementia can also be depressed and/or suffer from delirium. Obviously if one condition is superimposed on another condition, the person's abilities are further impaired.

A thorough diagnostic evaluation begins with a thorough medical and social history. This is best obtained from a reliable family member. It is important to know about general health, health of family members both dead and living, a picture of the present problem and any history of previous emotional disorders. Vision and hearing disorders must be identified and treated, as they may increase confusion in mental disorders. Finally, work history and education may also offer clues.

A mental status examination is an important part of the assessment. The person's orientation to time, place, person and season is obtained. Memory is tested for both recent and remote information. The examiner should be well-trained for this activity and be prepared to deal with the patient's stress when confronting very painful facts.

One way to evaluate recent memory is to use the three words at 5 minutes test. The patient is told three words, asked to repeat them and instructed to remember them for recall in 5 minutes. Remote memory can be tested by asking for significant dates such as birth, wedding, etc.

Reversibility is lost in dementia states. This is tested by having the patient spell a word forward and then backward. To test knowledge about general information, one can ask about opinions related to current events.

The patient should also have a neurologic examination which may help to identify certain characteristics of a brain lesion. It is also helpful to assess intelligence level, visual-spatial function, judgment, etc. Skull x-rays and computerized brain scanning are routinely done, and an electroencephalogram (EEG) is also used. Of course, no examination is complete without blood and urine laboratory analysis. Evaluation of all of these data will confirm some conditions and only indicate others such as Alzheimer's disease. However, even this so called "rule out" disease (because there is no specific test for it) is confirmed by autopsy in about 85 percent of the cases diagnosed prior to death.

Treatment and Management: The treatment of an irreversible dementing process is aimed at the provision of good basic personal care and attempts to manage behavior symptoms that may be detrimental to the patient. Safety and security are critical to accident prevention because of impaired judgment. These persons are often restless, have altered sleep cycles, pace, and wander. Use of restraints should be carefully planned based on individual assessment, rather than routine, because of the need for regular and frequent opportunity to exercise freely.

Another component of care is the need for stimulation through touch and speech. Because of serious speech problems, patients are often described as being totally unaware of their surroundings. This is unfortunate because patients with dementia are usually painfully aware that some catastrophic incident has occurred. They require a great deal of verbal input and it often helps to get their attention by gently touching the arm or hand. They also need an opportunity to try to communicate with whatever speech is available, no matter how laborious.

Patients with a dementia are often described as aggressive. This probably is not part of the disease. The patient may strike out, push staff or family, shout, etc. Close review of such incidents often reveals that a situation seemed frightening. Staff may only be trying to get the patient to go to the dining room. The patient with these difficulties may perceive this as dangerous, especially when staff try to push or pull with their hands. Some of these episodes also seem to occur when a patient is tired and when their environment is more stimulating than their coping abilities can handle. It takes a well-trained staff to prevent these episodes and/or to keep them from escalating to a "terrible fright," as one dementia patient explained.

MEDICAL SERVICES

The Minnesota Medical Association has identified the major areas of physician care for the aged. First of all, they say that active involvement of elderly patients is necessary in discussions of decisions to accept or refuse treatment to be consistent with the Patient's Bill of Rights. If the patient is not mentally competent, a family member or guardian must participate in such discussions. More specifically, physician responsibilities include:

• Providing quality health care as economically as possible.

• Recommending health promotion measures to maximize an active lifestyle and promote optimal function.

• Making an accurate diagnosis based on special knowledge of the aging process and disease processes.

• Providing ongoing medical evaluation and treatment of all conditions.

• Ensuring continuity and coordination of care.

• Facilitating good communications with the patient, the family, and caregivers.

• Discussing with the patient and family the nature and course of the disease and treatment alternatives.

• Supporting the patient in informed decision making regarding treatment and the use of life support technology.

Medical service in residential care settings is often minimal in spite of 1974 federal regulations mandating regular physician visits, medical directors, and utilization review committees in nursing homes. Elderly persons, their families, staff and community require physician participation because the elderly 1) have multiple diseases which interact with one another, 2) have multiple therapies which require monitoring, 3) have psychological problems that need attention, 4) need palliative care during terminal illness, and 5) need assistance in deciding when and how much treatment should be given.

If a physician does not perform his or her minimum duties as required by law, nursing homes, not the physicians, are responsible. This can become a very difficult situation. Therefore, administrators need to have assistance in determining what constitutes good medical care and how to go about upgrading quality of care throughout the organization. This is achieved through an active medical director who clearly identifies his/her major responsibilities.

THE MEDICAL STAFF

There are two basic models for organizing the medical staff of a nursing home. The first, the closed model, limits the number of attending physicians to only a few physicians or to "house doctors only." The second, the open model, allows most physicians in the service area to admit patients. The latter is the most common arrangement, but it is also the most difficult to manage for an administrator.

There is no incentive for a doctor who has an occasional resident, seen only once a month, to follow the protocol and policies of an organization. Therefore, some mechanism must be put in place to assure appropriate medical care. In many instances, the Utilization Review Committee serves as the governing body for the medical staff and helps to support the Medical Director who functions as a physician supervisor. In addition, some kind of Medical Practice Agreement should delineate the responsibilities and obligations of both the attending physician and the nursing home. The document should be signed by each admitting doctor who must at the same time present his credentials. Model contracts are available from the American Medical Director's Association, 1200 15th St. NW, Washington, DC 20004.

THE MEDICAL DIRECTOR

By law, the Medical Director is responsible for coordinating medical care to ensure the adequacy and appropriateness of patient medical services. This includes developing and implementing policies regarding primary physician credentialing, granting of staff privileges, compliance with regulations and disciplinary procedures.

The Medical Director must also develop policies regarding physician participation in the major committees; pharmacy, infection control, ethics, quality assurance, utilization review (UR), and safety. He or she will also be responsible for the mechanism to provide emergency services. It should be noted that some medical directors prefer to have no patients of their own where they serve in this position. This prevents any conflict of interest issues from rising.

There also needs to be policies regarding employee health. Should employees have a pre-employment physical examination? What should staff do when they have infections? What should an employee do when injured on the job?

In addition, general resident health needs must be considered. What measures should be taken when there is a community flu outbreak? If there is a pet in the residence, what health measures must be taken? What infection control measures are needed when a resident has an infection? What protocols are necessary to monitor resident falls and accidents?

The Medical Director's responsibility for education should be directed especially toward staff and physicians. For physicians, education may entail formal presentations at a medical conference or informal conferences on the telephone, in the hall, or at the bedside. For staff, regular patient rounds can be an excellent opportunity for informal teaching. These rounds can be combined with patient care, or be planned for teaching only. When disruptive resident behavior exhausts and frustrates staff, staff support will not only assist staff, but it will also help to generate better staff/resident relationships. More formal inservice education is ofcourse another teaching method.

ADMINISTRATOR RESPONSIBILITIES FOR MEDICAL CARE

The relationship of the medical director and the administrator must be based on mutual respect for one another's knowledge and responsibilities. It is critical that the Medical Director's personality be such that he or she has equal respect for the input of nurses, housekeepers, social workers and others who are involved in patient care and who see the resident on a daily basis. Health care in a residential setting is a team effort requiring all professional and non-professional staff, as well as families and residents themselves.

The administrator is responsible for recruiting a medical director who is both interested and competent in geriatric medicine. It is critical that this person's duties and responsibilities be identified in a contract. Some of the most critical responsibilities of the medical director include 1) development and monitoring of patient care policies and procedures, 2) development of policies and procedures regarding employee health, 3) regular review of data related to quality assurance, utilization, infection control, accidents, and drug use, 4) liaison with the medical community and intervention with physicians who are not in compliance with medical care standards and regulations, and 5) educational input for the entire organization. The administrator's role in finding and keeping a competent medical director is critical to the health care program of the organization.

RESOURCES FOR LONG-TERM MEDICAL CARE

Alzheimer's Disease & Related Disorders Association, Inc., (ADRDA) 8053 E. Bloomington Freeway, Bloomington, MN 55420 excellent resources

Anderson, Sir Ferguson and Brian Williams. *Practical Management of the Elderly.* 4th ed., St. Louis, MO, C. V. Mosby, 1984.

Conrad, Kenneth, Ed. *Drug Therapy for the Elderly.* St. Louis, MO, C. V. Mosby, 1982.

Cape, Ronald. *Aging: Its Complex Management.* New York, Harper and Row, 1978.

Haug, M. R. and M. Powell Lawton. *Elderly Patients and Their Doctors.* New York, NY, Springer Publishing, 1981.

Kane, R. A. and Kane, R. L. *Assessing the Elderly: A Practical Guide to Measurement.* Lexington, MA, Lexington Books, 1981.

Kane, R. L., Ouslander, J. G., and Abrass, I. *Essentials of Clinical Geriatrics.* New York, NY, McGraw-Hill, 1984.

Lehmann, J. D. "Health Care for the Elderly—A Minnesota Physician's Perspective," *Minnesota Medicine.* March 1985, pp. 224–233.

REFERENCES

Butler, Robert. "Geriatrics in Action: Getting Older and Getting Better," *Healthcare Executive,* 2:2:24–27, March/April, 1987.

Cape, Ronald. *Aging: Its Complex Management.* New York, Harper and Row, 1978.

Joint Commission on Accreditation of Hospitals. *Accreditation Manual for Long-Term Care Facilities.* Chicago, IL 1986.

Maletta, G. J. and Campion, M. E. "Behavior: A Symptom of Cognitive and

Functional Disorders" in Gordon, G.K. and Stryker, R., Ed. *Creative Long-Term Care Administration.* Springfield, IL, Charles C Thomas, 1st edition, 1983.

Mortimer, James A. et al. "Alzheimer's Disease: The Intersection of Diagnosis, Research, and Long-Term Care". PS Bulletin of the New York Academy of Medicine 61:5:331–342, May 1985.

Pattee, James. "Update on the Medical Director Concept," *The American Family Physician,* 28:6:129–133, 1983.

Rowe, John W. "Health Care of the Elderly," *New England Journal of Medicine.* 312:13:827–835, March 28, 1985.

Spilseth, Paul. *Medical Practice Agreement for Attending Physicians: A Model for Nursing Homes* and *Defining the Relationship: the Medical Director and Attending Physicians.* A project of the Minnesota Association of Medical Director's of Nursing Homes and the American Medical Directors Association, 1987.

Chapter 15

THE DEPARTMENT OF NURSING

Ruth Stryker

Approximately 60 percent of all personnel employed in a long-term care facility work in the nursing department. These direct care givers have the greatest amount of interaction with residents as well as families, especially during evenings and weekends. Because a long-term care facility builds its reputation on the quality of care rendered to its residents, it is critical that nursing staff have good communication skills and be clinically competent.

First, all RN's and LPN's must practice according to the Nursing Practice Act of the state or Canadian province of employment. Each Act defines the scope and limitations for licensed practice. Each employer must require visible evidence of current licensure of all RN's and LPN's annually. Second, every nursing department must meet its profession's standards by adhering to both the American Nurses' Association Standards for Organized Nursing Services and Gerontological Nursing Practice Standards.

The work of the nursing department is to provide residents with individualized care based on sound geriatric nursing knowledge. This means that each resident is reviewed in the following areas: 1) physical care and comfort, 2) environment and safety, 3) psychosocial needs, 4) intellectual stimulation, 5) maintenance and rehabilitative measures, and 6) prevention of nosocomial (institution acquired) illness. Each resident should be assessed for the level of function and the level of potential or susceptibility in all of these areas. The data gathered through this process forms a base for developing a nursing care plan.

PHILOSOPHY AND GOALS

The philosophy for the nursing department must be consistent with the institutional philosophy, interpreting basic premises into nursing directions. It must be in writing, and available to personnel, residents, and families. Philosophy statements often include such phrases as: respect

181

for the dignity and worth of the individual (care giver as well as resident), a home-like atmosphere, holistic approach, family participation in care, and helping the resident to achieve and maintain maximum independence. It is important to share the nursing philosophy with potential employees prior to confirming employment. All personnel within the department should be able to "buy in" to the philosophy and support it.

Goals and objectives are equally important for the department. These are more specific statements which again should flow from the institution's goals. They are usually written with a time frame for achievement. They should be reasonable and achievable for the stated time period. Ideally, they should be written prior to budget preparation so that they can be funded adequately. They should be approved by the administrator and can serve as a basic evaluation tool for the department.

THE ORGANIZATIONAL PLAN

The organizational plan for the department of nursing shows the relationships between nursing personnel and other departments. The plan should 1) allow the director of nursing direct access to the administrator, 2) allow efficient communication between key individuals, 3) permit decisions to be made at appropriate levels, and 4) clearly show lines of authority.

Clearly defined job descriptions for each category of personnel should include statements of major performance responsibilities. To assure that the performance evaluation flows directly from the job description, it is necessary to develop performance standards. For each major performance responsibility identified in the job description, an outcome statement is developed to indicate when performance is satisfactory. Next, the standards or components that make up satisfactory performance are identified.

For example, if a job description says "practices clinical nursing based on a sound knowledge of nursing practice," the performance is satisfactory when a nurse incorporates the nursing process while planning, organizing, directing, and controlling activities in the nursing unit. This achievement would be evident if the nurse makes resident assessment rounds, makes appropriate nursing care assignments, assesses the total unit function, participates in planning staffing, implements systems to carry out high quality nursing care, and evaluates the effectiveness of care systems and individual care.

POLICIES, PROCEDURES AND ROUTINES

Nursing care policies and procedures must be up-to-date through periodic review and revision. There are many excellent references available. Consequently, it is not necessary for nursing personnel to spend an inordinate amount of time writing procedures. It is important for staff members to have access to policies and procedures both on each nursing station and in the nursing office. A master index is useful to guide staff to the right resource.

Unfortunately, many institutional routines have been established for the convenience of care givers rather than residents. Granted, some activities must occur within certain time parameters such as breakfast between 7 and 9 AM and dinner between 5:30 and 6:30 PM to abide by state regulations specifying the amount of time between dinner and breakfast. However, rigid times are not necessary. Many other activities take place because of staffing patterns or institutional convenience rather than adapting to life-time patterns of residents. A good example of this is the ritual of settling residents for bed. This normally occurs sometime between 8:30 and 10:00 PM. Yet, it is a well-known fact that as people age, they require less sleep than younger persons and may not be ready to retire until after the night shift comes on duty.

QUALIFICATIONS OF NURSING PERSONNEL

In order to understand the nursing department, the administrator needs to be aware of the various educational levels of nursing staff to assure that care givers of different skill and knowledge not be used interchangeably. There are two categories of licensed nurses—the registered nurse (R.N.) and the licensed practical nurse (L.P.N.), in some states called the licensed vocational nurse (L.V.N.).

PROGRAMS FOR R.N.'s

Diploma Programs: Nursing education in the United States began as apprenticeship training in hospitals. The majority of all nurses in the U.S. have graduated from hospital schools of nursing and have been granted a diploma. Student nurses in these three-year programs had a significant amount of clinical experience. More recently, there has been greater emphasis on academic study than clinical experience. As a result, many hospital-based schools closed because they were unable to operate a financially viable educational program with this altered emphasis.

Associate Degree Program: Associate degree programs began in the two-year community colleges. These programs usually divide the two years between academic courses and clinical experience at a local hospital or nursing home. The limited amount of time in these programs naturally limits exposure to the clinical setting prior to graduation.

Baccalaureate Program: Baccalaureate nursing programs in four-year colleges or universities enable students to have a basic liberal arts background which includes greater knowledge of biological and psychosocial sciences than the shorter programs. Because of the heavy emphasis on academic preparation, clinical experience is also limited. However, students also spend time in a public health and mental health setting in addition to the more traditional assignments in hospitals and nursing homes.

The American Nurses' Association Committee on Education continues to attempt to set four major directions for basic nursing education:

1. All education for licensed nurses should take place in an institution of higher learning.
2. Minimum education for a beginning professional nurse should be a baccalaureate degree.
3. Minimum education for a beginning technical nurse should be an associate degree.
4. Education for assistants should be "short, intensive preservice programs in vocational education institutions rather than on-the-job training programs."

Postgraduate Programs: Most states have at least one college or university which offers an advanced degree in nursing. The major foci of the graduate programs are nursing administration, nursing education, or clinical nursing that includes specialties in geriatrics, psychiatry, public health, or maternal and child health. Graduates of masters programs usually find positions as highly qualified clinical specialists, faculty members, consultants or nursing administrators. There are a few doctoral level programs for nurses. Doctoral programs heavily emphasize the research component.

Other postgraduate courses are available through institutions of higher learning, such as nurse practitioner programs.

Nurse practitioners may be employed by a physician or healthcare organization, or they may be self-employed. While their responsibilities vary somewhat both within and among states, they generally provide a much needed link between patient and physician by giving direct services which include physical examination and assessment, health counselling and recommending diagnostic examinations and selected interventions based upon protocols mutually developed with physicians.

The nurse practitioner, an R.N. who has usually had one year of special education in the above areas, can make a very special contribution both to the nursing care and to the medical care of nursing home residents. Such a position can literally fill the gap caused by the minimal involvement of physicians in most nursing homes. He or she can quickly intervene when a resident's condition changes and initiate care. This is enabled by the collaborative work relationship that is developed with the physician.

When a nurse practitioner is introduced, it is crucial that the organization prepare its staff, especially the nursing staff, for this new role. This requires the help of the physician in order to carefully delineate the duties, responsibilities, and staff relationships of all concerned. Staff must understand the role, skills, authority and limitations of the nurse practitioner. In certain situations, the nurse practitioner deals more frequently and directly with nursing personnel than does the physician. The latter requires time and attention during the period of adjustment by the nursing staff to the altered communication pattern with physicians.

PROGRAMS FOR L.P.N.'s OR L.V.N.'s

The practical nurse is usually a graduate of a vocational or technical school of nursing. The program includes basic fundamentals of bedside care and clinical experience in a neighboring hospital and nursing home. This one-year educational program does not allow time for in-depth scientific principles to be included in the curriculum; therefore, it is understandable that state licensure laws require that the L.P.N. work under the direction of a registered nurse, physician or dentist. Upon successful completion of an L.P.N. program, the graduate is eligible to take a licensure examination. Successful completion of this examination enables the graduate to become a licensed vocational nurse (L.V.N.) or a licensed practical nurse (L.P.N.), whichever title is used by the state.

EDUCATION OF NURSE ASSISTANTS

A few states offer a three- to six-week nursing assistant training program through the vocational schools. There are also programs which train a nurse assistant to administer limited medications in a long-term care setting. Because nurse assistants give the major portion of patient care it is the responsibility of the director of nursing to differentiate the duties which can be legally performed by each category of care giver and assure that they are both adequately trained and supervised.

UTILIZATION OF NURSING PERSONNEL

Are R.N.'s under utilized? Are L.P.N.'s assigned tasks beyond their knowledge? Are L.P.N.'s and R.N.'s used interchangeably for the same assigned responsibilities? Are baccalaureate prepared R.N.'s used interchangeably with associate degree prepared R.N.'s? Are nursing assistants assigned patients with problems about which they know very little? Do nursing assistants lack adequate on-the-job training and supervision? Is resident care therapeutically oriented? The list of questions is of course endless, but they are commonly encountered situations in long-term care nursing.

RN/LPN UTILIZATION

Historically, hospitals have differentiated the job descriptions and assignments of R.N.'s and L.P.N.'s more clearly than nursing homes. The latter frequently assign R.N.'s and L.P.N.'s to identical responsibilities. The most important reason for this lack of delineation in nursing homes stems from the federal requirement of a "licensed" nurse on duty. This regulation not only fails to recognize the differences in nursing education, but it implies skill interchangeability, and suggests minimal resident needs.

In order to change this situation, one must begin with both the R.N. and L.P.N. job description. How do they differ and in what respects? It is this author's belief that 1) an organization cannot justify salary differentials between these two levels of nursing unless their work assignments differ, 2) residents should not lose the benefit of the R.N.'s highest skills, and 3) R.N. morale is weakened by equating their skill with that of an L.P.N.

In order to circumvent these problems, one must establish a hierarchy of skill complexity. Unfortunately, these positions are usually described in terms of tasks. For instance, both can make beds, but so can house-keeping personnel. Both can pass medications, but so can some nursing assistants. An endless list of tasks does not clarify the issue of role and function.

In a nursing home, the R.N. should be used at the highest skill level. This means that she assesses nursing needs, tries various approaches for improved physical and mental function, evaluates the effectiveness of intervention, assists personnel to carry out consistent care and participates in teaching other personnel. While she can do other things, the majority of her time should be spent in these areas.

The LPN is educated to provide physical and some rehabilitative care. Again, the organization should use her highest skills. When an LPN is assigned the same duties as the nursing assistant, nursing levels are again blurred. In order to avoid this, nursing assistants can be trained and assigned to personal care, assistance with bathing, grooming, dressing and eating. However, if the resident needs rehabilitation in these areas, the L.P.N. should be providing the care based on specific goal-oriented plans developed by the R.N.

From this kind of base, a director of nursing and her staff can begin to think in terms of developing job descriptions around job function and responsibilities rather than tasks. If the R.N. is to perform at the cognitive level for which she has been prepared, it means that she will give direct care to residents on a rotating basis. However, when she gives care, it is not to perform a necessary daily task. It is done to assess and upgrade the care assigned to others on future days. It should be done to develop new nursing interventions and to review the behavioral, rehabilitative and physical aspects of the care plan in depth. The L.P.N., on the other hand, should perform the more technical treatments and nursing measures and give care to persons with rehabilitation potential. Medications, foot care, decubitus care and heat treatments are examples.

Occasionally, an exceptionally capable L.P.N. works with an R.N. of similar skill. It is advisable not to have two such individuals working on the same unit. In the case of the R.N., every effort should be made to upgrade her skills. She might work more closely with another R.N. and the inservice director. She could be assigned specific readings and she might be encouraged to attend appropriate continuing education programs. If she cannot upgrade her skills to meet the requirements of the R.N. position, then she should not be allowed to remain in that position. In the case of the specially capable L.P.N., she needs to be given opportunity to use her talents. If she cannot return to school to become an R.N., she can be allowed to help with orienting new staff, provide a role model for other L.P.N.'s, work closely with residents with special problems and/or work on special committees. Her work surely deserves special recognition. In other words, job descriptions must clearly distinguish between positions, but allow for appropriate rewards for excellence.

WHO'S IN CHARGE?

The R.N.-L.P.N. issue also relates to the matter of the "charge" nurse. Nursing education programs are based on different levels of knowledge and skill related to patient conditions and needs, not on administrative skill. However, many employment settings expect administrative duties to be performed and reward charge duties either subtly or directly. This encourages nurses to seek administrative responsibility for psychological and/or monetary reasons without preparation.

Because two-thirds of the nursing staff of a nursing home is comprised of nursing assistants, scarce licensed personnel are required to work in some administrative capacity rather frequently. For some staff, this means caring for patients (being supervised) one day and being a supervisor the next. Such a situation leads to ineffectual supervision and strained interpersonal relations. L.P.N.'s like to work in nursing homes because they have "more responsibility," which usually means that they have access to "charge" responsibilities. Even when additional pay is not at issue, there is a sense of greater status and self-esteem when one does not take care of patients directly.

Every organization must decide what is required of a "charge" nurse and **then** decide who should do it. The job must be examined so that the question, "in charge of what?" is answered. Telephone calls to M.D.'s and the families? Calling the maintenance man to replace a light bulb? Giving directions to visitors? Giving medications? Finding replacement personnel? While our governmental regulations require a licensed person on duty, they do not necessarily mean "in charge". The intent is of course to have a qualified person available for nursing care. However, only some "charge" duties actually relate to nursing care. Once the duties of the "charge" person, particularly on relief and nights, differentiates the need for nursing skills from those of a receptionist, it will be far easier to decide who is needed. As a general rule, "charge" persons maintain the work flow during a particular time frame. They are not managers in the broad view, but they must coordinate communications and a team of workers for a shift. Therefore, communications skills and interpersonal skills are crucial. It may well be that a receptionist is the best person to be "in charge," freeing an R.N. to supervise the work of personnel, to monitor the condition of residents and to act in emergency situations.

Because the composition of a home's nursing staff, the size of patient units, and the level(s) of care vary so widely, it is only possible to suggest guidelines for approaching this problem.

1. The R.N. is the highest skilled person on your staff. In the case of a large organization, multiple levels of care or many skilled residents, at least one R.N. should be "in charge" of all resident/family care decisions. With this back-up, L.P.N.'s may work very satisfactorily at the unit "charge" level.

2. "Charge" nurses should be relieved of as many clerical and receptionist tasks as possible. A good rule of thumb is "when over 50 percent of a charge nurse's time is not related to direct care of residents and families, other kinds of personnel should be considered."

3. All "charge" nurses should be selected for and given special training in (a) organization of work, (b) interpersonal skills, (c) coaching effectively, (d) handling of emergencies, and (e) the importance of uniform performance expectations.

4. "Charge" persons should be stable full time personnel whenever possible. If this is impossible, selected persons should be regularly assigned to "charge" duties to reduce frequently changing "bosses" who have little influence on their job status and often have different performance expectations. In addition, some personnel behave much like a student when there is a substitute teacher. This is unfair to residents as well as the charge person.

5. "Charge" assignments must not allow one employee to supervise another employee one day and then reverse the roles the next. Such peer supervision is fraught with potential problems.

6. Evaluation of personnel who work straight relief or nights must be assigned to someone who works regularly with them and is trained in this task.

7. "Charge" nurses must of course be specifically evaluated for their "charge" function.

R.N./L.P.N./N.A. RATIOS

During the past decade many hospitals have altered the mix of their nursing staff by increasing the numbers of R.N.'s and L.P.N.'s and decreasing the numbers of nursing assistants. Those who have done this report an improved use of staff time as well as a higher grade of care. In some instances, staff costs have been reduced or remained about the same, depending upon the internal ratio changes.

Jelinek found that at one medical center nursing assistants had an unusually large amount of unoccupied time. This idle or so-called down time averaged about 27 percent each day. This means in effect that every fourth aide was unoccupied due to a limited range of duties caused by minimal training. In other words, one may not necessarily have to make a one for one replacement. Three L.P.N.'s might conceivably replace four nursing assistants. It should be noted that this does not result in more work for the L.P.N.'s.

Christman and others found the same phenomenon. He found that when the ratio of licensed personnel to nursing assistants was virtually reversed, the turnover rate went down and the stability rate went up. In addition, the cost of orientation and education time was reduced because of fewer nursing assistants who require so much on-the-job training and supervision.

This idea should not be dismissed by nursing home administrators. Because of the impact on cost, turnover and quality of care, various mixes of nursing personnel should be seriously studied and tried in every home. It may even vary between nursing units. While the number of staff per patient has importance, the mix of the staff may be even more important. One nursing home unit uses all R.N.'s with a reduction of four positions.

At another nursing home the administrator decided to apply this idea to his 125-bed organization. He decided to proceed cautiously. Over a three-month period, he replaced nine nursing assistant positions with seven L.P.N. positions. He did this as natural attrition of nursing assistants occurred. The cost of this change was one penny per patient day.

The effect of this change was felt almost immediately. The inservice director found time to plan more creative programming because she was released from constant repetitive teaching of new aides. Favorable comments on the quality of care from residents and families increased. Staff commented on greater work satisfaction because of improved care of residents. While this particular administrator made several changes aimed at reducing turnover in his organization, he felt this action contributed significantly to its reduction. He believed the latter was due to the interrelationship of improved work satisfaction, improved client satisfaction, fewer interruptions due to questions from less trained personnel, less dissatisfaction about the kind of care being delivered and a greater overall pride in the organization.

The Benedictine Nursing Center in Mt. Angel, Oregon, looked at nursing staff mix, and decided to substitute a nursing assistant position for an R.N. position. The administrator reports a marked decrease in the use of drugs (as demonstrated by a decrease in drug costs and recording on resident records), a significant number of persons who used to use wheelchairs are now walking, a decrease in the number of incontinent patients and markedly fewer family complaints.

Work sampling of actual use of time by nursing personnel is the most accurate way of making management decisions about changing the mix of nursing staff. However, a cautious and gradual change which is carefully monitored may be a very realistic way of beginning. If seven L.P.N.'s can replace nine nursing assistants for one penny a patient day, could thirteen L.P.N.'s replace eighteen nursing assistants at a cost reduction? While cost should not be the primary concern, certainly finding ways of upgrading care within cost constraints needs to be explored more creatively than they have to date. Some administrators are finding ways of doing both.

Until very recently, attention to productivity was thought to be a problem of the business world, certainly not a concern of those of us in human services! However, this immunity from examining productivity has come to an abrupt end. The cost of health care is under close scrutiny of peers, government, tax payers, insurance companies, health care providers and health care recipients. If one looks at this list of interested parties, you will see that "we" and "they" are the same. As Pogo said, "We have met the enemy and they are us."

The challenge of today's health care administrator is to provide the best possible care without further escalation of costs. One way is to examine worker productivity. What is even more surprising, is that quality of care can often be improved at the same time. Certainly the employment of fewer untrained personnel who turn over frequently because they become discouraged, because they are expected to work at a level beyond their knowledge and training, and who spend as much time being trained as they do working, is a step in the right direction. Attention to productivity of personnel can provide impetus to changes that may also result in reduced employee turnover. Altering the mix of nursing staff is but one example.

METHODS OF ASSIGNING NURSING STAFF

One method of nursing assignment is team nursing. Under this system, eight to twenty patients, depending upon their conditions, are assigned to two or more nursing staff usually of different educational levels. One of the most frequently cited problems with this system is that the team mix constantly changes because of days off. This violates knowledge about interpersonal behavior for effective group function. In addition, it requires some management training which few nurses have. Neither does it take into account individual differences. It assumes that any R.N. is capable of being a team leader.

Another method of assignment is modular nursing which assigns nurses to geographical areas of patients. While this saves steps and eases the task of making assignments, it does not necessarily guarantee the right staff person with the right resident. It does have the advantage of assigning residents to fewer personnel. Team nursing and modular nursing can obviously go hand in hand and often do.

Functional assignments are quite efficient in getting the work done, but they divide the patient into artificial parts by assigning medications to one person, treatments to another, baths to another etc. The opposite method of assignment is called the total care or case method which assigns one person to all of the care for one patient. This has a tendency to either under- or over-utilize many members of the nursing staff.

All of these systems have one common deficiency; namely, a different staff person is responsible for a patient every eight hours and no one is accountable for the overall care and ultimate outcomes. Primary nursing overcomes this problem. A primary nurse is assigned to a patient for whom he or she is accountable for twenty-four hours from the time of admission through discharge and its attending plans. Other major elements of primary nursing include the coordination of nursing care with other disciplines, participation of both the patient and the family, careful assessment of care plans, encouraging communication of care givers and correction of care givers when necessary.

This twenty-four-hour versus eight-hour accountability enables the resident to identify with one nurse who is answerable for his or her total care. The patient/resident knows who this person is and benefits from realizing that nursing care is not just a matter of receiving pills, hot packs and denture care. Other personnel obviously give direct care when the primary nurse is not on duty, but the accountable person never changes.

Primary nursing has been used occasionally in nursing homes. Sister Mary Schwab has described its use at the Benedictine Nursing Center in Oregon. Here, the emphasis is on patient care which is not synonymous with "aide work." Primary nurses are R.N.'s who coordinate nursing care with other therapies, conduct interdisciplinary conferences, assess and evaluate the outcomes of interventions and work with families. If personnel on other shifts do not agree with the primary nurse's care plan orders, they leave a note or call her about their observations and concerns. Ward clerks are used for paperwork and other tasks that are essential to enabling nurses to provide care. Depending on the intensity of needs, one R.N. may be the primary nurse for as many as twenty residents or as few as five.

One Minnesota nursing home has adapted primary nursing to include L.P.N.'s and nursing assistants. This enables the home to recognize the special capabilities of selected L.P.N.'s and nursing assistants. While an R.N. periodically reviews all residents, the primary care person (1) regularly reports the physical, social and behavioral function of residents to families, (2) reports any changes immediately to families, and (3) uses families for input to care plans. Families know which staff person has the most information about their relative. Patients assigned to primary nursing assistants are usually stabilized and receive a minimum number of medications and treatments. Those assigned to primary L.P.N.'s require a greater number of medications, treatments and rehabilitation measures. New admissions and those with complex physical and behavioral problems are assigned to R.N.'s.

Primary nursing requires special commitment and knowledge that does not just happen by fiat. All staff must be introduced to the concept. Those administering it must be introduced to the concept. Those administering it must be introduced to the concept. Those administering it must study the subject to prevent the predictable pitfalls experienced by those who do not think through its effect on all departments. Those who carry out the role of the primary nurse must be prepared to do it well. The readings at the end of this chapter have been selected to assist nursing directors to understand how to make primary nursing a dynamic method of upgrading care. Its ultimate effect on morale and pride in outcomes relates directly to many of the research issues described in Part III.

PERSONAL CONSIDERATIONS OF STAFF

The relationship between turnover rates, staff preference, possible burnout from constant work with heavy care patients, and the complexity of patient problems encountered by new employees must be addressed. A new employee, especially the nursing assistant, seems to prefer working with the less disabled during the first few months when the greatest learning is taking place. Working with these residents provides both experience and learning that can serve as an introduction to working with the more disabled. It also helps to reduce the sense of anxiety and helplessness so often described by new employees who resign after only a few weeks or months on the job. This, coupled with the suggestions for orientation and supervision of the new employee in Chapter 11 can help to minimize many of these problems.

Burnout, the emotional and physical drain that accompanies many jobs in human services is widely recognized in mental health, chemical dependency, special education, hospice care and other fields. This phenomenon has received far less attention in geriatric services. Management needs to determine organizational practices that perpetuate it. Some nursing homes plan intermittent discussion groups with a social worker or psychologist to deal with these feelings. Other homes rotate staff between heavy care and lesser care units. Unfortunately, this practice is often done on a regular basis for all employees rather than on an individual basis. Routine rotation of all staff between levels of care is far more disruptive (both to residents and employees) than when it is done on request by an individual.

Nursing departments must also consider individual differences that relate to work satisfaction. Some nursing home personnel receive greater satisfaction from working with severely disabled patients while others prefer to work with the less disabled. Such choices should be honored in staff placements whenever possible. If an individual prefers to care for severely disabled persons, because they feel "more needed," it could enhance dependency and impede any rehabilitation potential or improved self-esteem. Inservice programming can help to channel these motivations into more therapeutic behaviors.

Administrators must also be cognizant of negative rewards. We must be aware that the person who writes care plans well is often the person who ends up writing most of the care plans; likewise, the person who is willing to work an extra shift gets called most often. Because of these factors, nurses feel exploited unless we build ways to allow them to teach skills to others and thereby share the responsibility and work load.

SCHEDULING NURSING HOURS

Both policies and systems for scheduling personnel hours are frequently non-existant in nursing homes. Matching a name with a shift does not take into account staff's need to plan for personal affairs, the physiological effect of constantly changing shifts, and the impact of these matters on the quality of care to residents.

Police, firemen, and people who work at restaurants and hotels are valuable resources for well-thought out systems. The following synthesize the preparation for a sound scheduling system.

Analysis of Present System: Who prepares hour schedules? Is this the appropriate person? Should the department head do it? How many persons are doing it? Can someone else be trained to do it better? Do personnel work too many days in a row? Are days off split or consecutive? When do personnel find out their work schedule—a few days, a week, two weeks, a month or three months in advance?

Analysis of Personnel Needs: What fluctuations occur in the work load— times of the day, evening or night and on what days of the week? How do peaks in the work load affect the quality of performance, absenteeism and fatigue? How many persons have idle time, at what hours, for how long?

Developing a Plan

The organization must first ask the right questions. Can work schedules be made more flexible to fit with today's lifestyles? What about job sharing? Would more part time staff provide more effective coverage for care? Would the 4-day work week be helpful?

The best way to begin a plan is to leave out the names of present personnel and to ignore the staffing schedule in current use. Using graph paper, write in the number and level of staff required for every 2-hour period. You will quickly note fluctuations. From this, you may well determine new staffing patterns such as overlap of shifts, new shifts, part shifts, etc.

Remember, the objective of this exercise is to develop staffing needs based on work loads. Can some work be back logged or changed to a different time or be done by someone else? Do not let yourself revert to the present system. Be creative. Once this is done, selected employees should review the plan and provide ideas for modification. Once this is completed, you have a basic design for one-week which can then be translated to a 4-, 6- or 8-week schedule.

The nursing department has the best reason to develop a master schedule because they provide round-the-clock coverage seven days a week. For decades head nurses have "made out hours" weekly. It was an extra job, usually postponed to the end of the week, resulting in staff who did not know when they would work until the Friday of the week before the schedule. The reason police and firemen complain less about their hours is because they know them well in advance so they can plan their personal lives.

Staffing secretaries are employed in many health care organizations. Aside from saving nursing time, this has the advantage of having someone other than the "boss" do it. Frequently, if a nurse has not performed well, she may imagine or actually find her hours less desirable than those who perform better. In any case, preparing nursing schedules is an administrative function, not a nursing function.

Preparing a four-week hour schedule takes very little more time than for a one-week schedule. In addition, staff will be appreciative. For example, if a friend calls someone to play bridge next Thursday night, s/he will know whether it is possible. She can either suggest another night or trade hours with someone in the same job category.

Once a four-week schedule is prepared, it can almost be duplicated every four weeks. This nearly identical staffing distribution is called "cyclical staffing" or "master staffing." While it takes time to develop a master schedule the first time, it saves many hours in the long run.

Flexible Scheduling

There will be increasing competition for nurses in the coming decade. This competition will be intensified by a growing shortage of nurses mainly caused by 1) an increased variety of occupations open to women, 2) a decreasing number of persons in the age group entering college, and 3) a greater variety and number of new nursing positions. Therefore new ideas are needed.

If an organization resorts to frequent reliance on outside personnel pools, regular staff are forced to work less popular shifts. To counter this situation, a home may set up its own pool. There are other ways such as flexible scheduling.

Flexible scheduling does not mean abandoning master staffing plans, it means working such persons into a master plan. It does not mean that someone can dictate their hours at a moment's notice. It means that new and more creative personnel systems are required, including greater flexibility in terms of the traditional shifts as shown in Figure 15-1.

One hospital has worked out a very interesting set of shift and hour combinations that has helped to keep nursing staff who were not satisfied with traditional work hours. Here are the choices given personnel all of whom have every other weekend off. Full-time RN and LPN options—work days with EITHER rotation to nights or relief, permanent evenings or nights, may work 8-, 10- or 12-hour shifts, may work 8-hour day shifts or 10-hour night shifts, may be assigned as a float or to a permanent station. Part-time options—may work a 5-, 8-, 10- or 12-hour shift, assigned to unit of choice when there is an opening.

Pool employees must work 16 hours a month, one weekend day a month and one holiday a year on any shift.

Flexible scheduling means just that. It does not mean that everyone must go to a nontraditional shift. One position might be filled by a person working from 7 AM to 5 PM, someone working from 5 PM to 9 PM and a third person who works 9 PM to 7 AM. Another position may be filled by persons working traditional shifts. The combinations are infinite if staff look at the work load and plan accordingly. In addition, the customary starting hours for shifts need not be rigid. Why can't someone come to work at 8 AM or 9 AM if some of our typical routines are altered? Experimenting with flexible staffing is both a challenge and a step toward obtaining and retaining staff who might not otherwise be in the work force or who might otherwise be in someone else's work force.

THE DIRECTOR OF NURSING

The director of nursing should be a registered professional nurse with managerial skills and preferably hold a baccalaureate degree. The person who holds this title should be carefully chosen and should be viewed as an essential member of the top management team for the facility. The long-term care administrator, the chief financial officer and the

4-WEEK HOUR SCHEDULE
Jan. 4–31 Station 3 B

	4 Su	5 M	6 T	7 W	8 Th	9 F	10 Sa	11 Su	12 M	13 T	14 W	15 Th	16 F	17 Sa	18 Su	19 M	20 T	21 W	22 Th	23 F	24 Sa	25 Su	26 M	27 T	28 W	29 Th	30 F	31 Sa
R.N.—Head nurse	7	7	0	7	7	H	0	0	7	7	7	0	7	7	7	7	0	7	7	9	0	0	7	7	7	0	7	7
R.N.—Team leader	0	7	7	0	7	7	7	7	0	7	3	7	7	0	0	3	3	0	3	0	3	7	0	7	7	7	H	0
R.N.—Team leader	3	7	7	7	3	7*	0	0	3*	3	0	3	H	3	3	0	7	7	7	H	0	0	7	3	0	7	7	3
R.N.—Team leader	0	3	3	3	0	3	3	3	7	0	7	7	0	0	3	7	7	3	0	7	7	7	3	0	3	3	3	0
L.P.N.	9	7	0*	7	7	9	0	0	3	3	3	3	0	9	9	7	7*	0	7	9	0	0	3	3	3	3	0	9
L.P.N.	0	3	3	3	3	0	9	9	7	7	0	7	9	0	0	3	3	3	3	0	9	9	7	7	0	7	9	0
Nursing assistant	7	0	0	7	7	7	0	0	7	7	7	7	7	3	3	0	0	7	7	7*	0	0	3	3	7	7	7	7
Nursing assistant	0	7	7	7	7	0	7	7	7	7	7	0	0	0	0	7	7	7	0	0	7	7	7	7	7	7	7	0
Nursing assistant	3	7	7	7	7	7	0	0	3	3	7	0	0	7	7	7	7	7	7	7	0	0	7	7	7	0	7	3
Nursing assistant	0	3	3	3	3	3	3	3	0	0	3	3	3	0	0	3	3	3	3	3	3	3	0	0	3	3	3	0
Station assistant	7	7	7	7	7	0	0	0	7	7	7	7	7	7	7	7	7	7	7	7	0	0	0	7	7	7	0	7
Station assistant	0	0	3	3	3	3	3	3	3	3	3	3	3	0	0*	0*	3	3	3	0	3	3	3	3	3	3	3	3
Station assistant—PT	3	3				3	0	0	3				3	3	3	3				3	0	0					7	3
Station assistant—PT	0						7	7	7				0	0						7	7	7	7					0

*Staff requests

Figure 15-1. Completed four-week hour schedule for all personnel on one nursing unit.

director of nursing must function in concert for a well-run organization.

The director has three managerial hats to wear: managing resident care, managing human resources, and managing supplies and equipment. Therefore, it stands to reason that the director be involved in organizational planning and budgeting.

The director of nursing for a long-term care facility is responsible for planning the care delivery system, establishing the standards of care (in keeping with the facility's mission statement), recruiting and retaining staff, providing for staff development and inservice education, and conducting ongoing quality assessments to assure that the care rendered is consistent with standards set. The director is responsible for establishing a philosophy of resident care, policies and procedures which are consistent with the kind of care provided, job descriptions for each category of care giver, performance evaluations which are criteria based and a care delivery system which is effective and efficient. In addition, the director has an important public relations role to play with residents, their families and friends, community groups, and referral agencies. The person in this position must also function as a resident advocate and establish collegial relationships with the medical staff and other allied health professionals.

The director must be thoroughly familiar with all state and federal regulations which govern resident care. From this broad knowledge base, the director assures that the care delivery system and the record keeping comply with those regulations. Because of the significant role that the director plays in a long-term care facility, the support of the long-term care administrator cannot be overemphasized.

SUMMARY

The nursing department is certainly the largest, and perhaps the most complex department in a nursing home. The management of this department demands an inquiring mind and a person who is willing to depart from the "old ways." This chapter has attempted to suggest some of these possibilities; namely, utilization of R.N.'s and L.P.N.'s, R.N./L.P.N./N.A. ratios, scheduling hours, the "charge" nurse, primary nursing, nurse practitioners, and attention to individual differences among employees. Certainly the director will develop additional ideas of her own as she searches for ways of improving the quality of life of elderly residents.

Recommended Resources for the Director of Nursing

Nursing Administration

Blake, Robert R., et al. *Grid Approaches for Managerial Leadership in Nursing.* St. Louis, MO, C.V. Mosby, 1981.

Creighton, Helen. *Law Every Nurse Should Know.* 4th ed., Philadelphia, W. B. Saunders, 1981.

Hoffman, Frances. *Financial Management for Nurse Managers.* E. Norwalk, CT., Robert J. Brady, 1983.

Hogstel, Mildred. *Management of Personnel in Long Term Care.* Bowie, M., Robert J. Brady, 1983.

Mauksch, I. and Miller, M. *Implementing Change in Nursing.* St. Louis, MO, C. V. Mosby, 1980.

Stevens, Barbara J. *The Nurse as Executive.* Wakefield, MA, Human Resources, 2nd ed., 1980.

Inservice Education

Ernest, Nora and West, Helen. *Nursing Home Staff Development, A Guide for Inservice Programs.* New York, Springer, 1983.

Kinney, Mark. *Staff Development in Geriatric Institutions.* Ann Arbor, MI, Institute of Gerontology, 1976.

Minninger Foundation. *Toward Understanding Therapeutic Care: A Training Guide for Inservice Education in the Psychosocial Components in L.T.C.* HCFA/HSQB, 1978, Superintendent of Documents, Washington, DC 20402.

Gerontological Nursing

Burnside, Irene M. *Working with the Elderly: Group Process and Techniques.* Monterey, CA, Wadsworth Health Sciences, 2nd ed., 1984.

Ebersole, Priscilla and Hess, Patricia. *Toward Healthy Aging.* St. Louis, MO, C. V. Mosby, 1981.

Flaherty, Maureen O'Brien. *The Care of the Elderly Person: A Guide for the Licensed Practical Nurse.* St. Louis, MO, C. V. Mosby, 1981.

Ragan, Pauline. *Aging Parents.* Los Angeles, Andrus Gerontology Center, 1979.

Simonson, William. *Medications and the Elderly.* Rockville, MD, Aspen Systems Corp., 1984.

Smith, Genevieve. *Care of the Patient with a Stroke.* New York, Springer, 2nd ed., 1976.

Steffl, Bernita, Ed. *Handbook of Gerontological Nursing.* New York, NY, Van Nostrand Reinhold, 1984.

Stryker, Ruth. *Rehabilitative Aspects of Acute and Chronic Nursing.* Philadelphia, W. B. Saunders, 2nd ed., 1977.

Wolanin, Mary Opal and Philips, Linda. *Confusion: Prevention and Care.* St. Louis, MO, C. V. Mosby, 1981.

Yurick, Ann, et al. *The Aged Person and the Nursing Process.* Norwalk, CT, Appleton-Century-Crofts, 2nd ed., 1984.

Journals

Geriatric Nursing
Journal of Gerontological Nursing
Journal of Nursing Administration
Rehabilitation Nursing

REFERENCES

Christman, Luther, "A Micro-Analysis of the Nursing Division of One Medical Center," in Millman, Michael, *Nursing Personnel and the Changing Health Care System*, Cambridge, Mass., Ballinger Publishing, 1977, pp. 143–152.

Golightly, Cecelia, "The Role of the Nursing Department," in Gordon, George K. and Ruth Stryker, Ed. *Creative Long-Term Care Administration*, Springfield, IL, Charles C Thomas, 1983.

Jelinek, R. et al., "A Structural Model for the Patient Care Operation," *Health Services Research*, 2:3 (Fall–Winter 1976).

Manthey, Marie, *The Practice of Primary Nursing*, London, Blackburn, 1980.

Schwab, Sister Marilyn, "Where Nurses' Aides Don't Do All the Nursing Care," *Journal of Gerontological Nursing*, May, June 1976, pp. 20–23.

Chapter 16

SOCIAL SERVICES IN LONG-TERM CARE

JOAN ABRAHAMSON

Social services are the major contributors to the psychosocial aspects of long-term care organizations. They will be discussed in terms of 1) the social work profession in long-term care, 2) direct social services to residents and families, 3) indirect services within the organization and community, and 4) administering social services.

THE SOCIAL WORK PROFESSION IN LONG-TERM CARE

This author takes an integrated approach to the health care of the individual, the family, the community, and the institution itself. As a holistic system, it aims to integrate and maximize physical, psychological, social, spiritual and environmental aspects of well-being. All individuals participate in and are responsible for their own health based on individual capacities. Social work has established methodologies in accordance with its professional 1) values, 2) ethics, 3) knowledge base, and 4) roles.

Social work values are based on humanistic and democratic ideals. Social services focus on utilization of resources. This includes the interaction between people and the social environment, the ways people interact with the informal systems of family and friends and the formal systems of health and social agencies. Minahan and Pincus (1977) describe these underlying values for social work practice as follows:

1. People should have access to the resources they need to accomplish life tasks, alleviate distress and realize their own aspirations and values.
2. The transactions between people of securing and utilizing resources should enhance their dignity, individuality, and self-determination.
3. These values should be the mutual responsibility of the individual citizen and collective society. Society's responsibility includes fostering conditions whereby citizens have opportunities to dis-

charge their social responsibilities to each other and to participate in the democratic process.

The ethical base of the profession is provided by the National Association of Social Workers Code of Ethics. This code establishes the conduct of the worker in relation to the client, colleagues, employer, the social work profession, and society. While the primary responsibility is to the client (maximize self-determination, respect privacy, and maintain confidential information), the social worker must also adhere to commitments made to the employing organization.

The social worker's knowledge base lies in human behavior and needs; social and emotional health problems; the psychological, social, economic, and physical effects of aging, illness, and disability; family and community systems and resources; and interactions between individuals and the social environment. The social worker's approach assumes that people can grow and change and that they can be helped to resolve their own problems and to cope with their environment.

Coulton (1981) and Monk (1981) have outlined the following social work objectives for the fields of health care and aging in general:

Help people enlarge competence; increase problem-solving and coping abilities.
Help people obtain resources.
Make organizations responsive to people.
Facilitate interactions between individuals and others in their environment.
Influence interactions between organizations and institutions.
Influence social and environmental policy.

These broad objectives for social work are appropriate to any long-term care service that assists the aged ill to function at maximum capacities.

The role of the social worker can be described most generally as that of a facilitator. This is accomplished through more specific roles: **interviewer**, collecting and giving information; **diagnostician**, making social assessments; **therapist/counselor**, providing individual and family counseling or therapy on a group or individual basis; **case manager**, providing interagency coordination of services; and (in long-term care) **transition manager**, a role that may combine all of the above roles in the process of relocation.

Underlying all social work roles is the role of **advocate**, assuring basic human and patient rights; and the role of **educator**, providing training and information to residents, their families, staff, and community. Other basic roles are those of **group worker,** working with residents and families in formal and informal groups; **community liaison and resource developer,** providing a linkage with community resources and helping to develop needed resources; **policy developer,** helping to develop policies and programs in the nursing home and in the community; **team member,** planning and implementing care, and collaborating and coordinating with staff; and **administrator,** planning, organizing, and directing social services.

DIRECT SOCIAL SERVICES TO RESIDENTS AND FAMILIES

Admission Services

Preadmission Services

Services during the preadmission period can be crucial in alleviating negative effects of relocation. Time must be allowed for social workers to assist applicants and families. In order to do this, many homes have successfully changed their policies to make time available. Essential services include the following:

1. Exposing the applicant and family to the nursing home environment. Whenever possible, applicants and families tour the facility, meet staff and other residents, observe activities and programs, and meet the roommate. If an applicant is hospitalized, the social worker and a nurse make a preadmission visit to the hospital. A photo album and an admissions booklet can help the applicant to visualize the nursing home. This can increase environmental predictability. Control can increase with discussion of preparations.

2. Conducting a personal interview with the applicant and family either in the home or hospital to provide and gather information. Honest information is given regarding the home, its policies, programs, routines, services, staffing, charges, and ways in which it might meet needs of the applicant. Questions and concerns of the applicant and family can be discussed honestly to lessen fears and anxieties. Such an interview helps both the applicant and the family to make an appropriate decision.

   Information is also gathered from family or significant others, hospital staff, or community agencies regarding the applicant's special needs, diagnosis, physical and mental functioning, social and emotional functioning, need for financial assistance, prior support systems, and attitudes and expectations of applicant and family towards the move. This information is used to assess the most appropriate decision for the applicant. If admission is decided upon, the information is used to plan initial care.

3. Establishing a supportive relationship. The worker-client relationship is the foundation for social services and is consciously developed. Because it is a helping and trust relationship, it can be undermined and cause conflicts if the social worker is asked to collect bills for the nursing home, or intervene in other inappropriate situations.

4. Counseling applicant and family with emphasis on a supportive relationship focuses on three main areas:
   a. Decision-making. Intervention may be needed to help the family to include the applicant wherever feasible in the decision-making process in order to maintain a sense of control.
   b. Helping the client to cope with the move. The social worker can help manage the crisis by maintaining supports already in place, encouraging open expressions of anger, and helping the individual to work through feelings of rejection and abandonment.
   c. Helping families to deal with the client's resentment and anger without being overwhelmed with guilt. Counseling can help families to cope with their feelings, maintain relationships, and support the person entering the nursing home.

5. Planning and preparing. Individualized planning and preparation for the move involves the active participation of the applicant as well as the family. This includes deciding what to do about previous living arrangements, personal belongings, and financial and legal matters. If needed, application for financial assistance is begun, admission papers signed, personal and property rights explained. Plans to bring personal items and to personalize the new environment are discussed. Admission procedures are explained and the day and time of admission are set.

6. Offering supportive services (legal, social, homemaker or health services) while waiting for admission.

7. Preadmission care planning. Information is shared with staff to prepare initial plans to meet the person's individual needs. In some homes this is done at an admission conference.

Both preadmission and admission practices are based on research results from studies on relocation which have identified factors that affect the impact of relocation. Among these factors the most noted are the degree of perceived control, the degree of environmental change, the degree of individualized planning and preparation, and the physical and mental health status of the individual (Bourestrom and Tars, 1974; Pablo, 1977; Lieberman, 1974; Bourestrom, Tars, Pastalan, 1974). Relocation is likely to have adverse effects if the move is forced, the environmental change is radical, there is little or no preparation for the move, and the individual is in poor health. However, if the individual can 1) maintain some control over the decision to move, 2) predict the environment, 3) cope with the discontinuity, participate in plans for the move and 4) has stabilized health, the move may, in fact, improve the health and functioning of the individual.

Environmental factors that produce a positive outcome have also been identified. They include providing a high degree of autonomy, placing more control in the hands of the resident, and setting high expectations for behavior. The environment can provide opportunities for privacy, constructive activities, social interaction, and access to the community. Staff must also treat residents as adults respecting their attitudes and accepting their ideas.

Personal characteristics of the individual are also powerful predictors of the outcome of relocation. The degree of hopelessness and despair was found to be the single most powerful predictors. Those who took a passive stance died at rates three times as great as those who took a more aggressive stance (Lieberman, 1974 and Tobin and Lieberman (1976).

Social services will attempt to minimize the negative effects of relocation and to maximize the individual's ability to adapt to the losses associated with the move and the new environment. Goals for admitting services are as follows:

Limit the amount of environment change.
Increase the amount of environmental predictability.
Increase the amount of control by the individual.
Provide active participation in planning and preparation.
Offer support and resources to maintain physical and mental health status.
Encourage development of attitudes and responses supportive of the move.
Limit number and accumulation of losses.

Admission to the Home

The social worker provides continuity and reassurance by welcoming the new resident and family on admission. Initial orientation may be limited to immediate surroundings and people because of fatigue and anxiety. The social worker and nurse explain admission procedures and help the resident settle in, physically and emotionally. Time is spent with the resident and family, listening to feelings and concerns, helping them cope with the immediate move, and completing any preadmission details.

Adjustment of the New Resident

Social services initially concentrate on reducing the traumatic effects of the move and facilitating the resident's adjustment. This is critical during the first three months, the time of highest morbidity and death rates. Residents are seen daily for the first week, then not less than twice a week, depending on the resident's needs. Besides working with individuals, social workers also meet with new residents and families in a group, together or separately. Additional support is, of course, necessary if families or significant others are not available.

Services during this period will concentrate on factors that promote adjustment.

1. Welcoming and orienting the new resident and family will include other residents, volunteers and staff. Welcoming parties, special recognition, and special orientation groups for new residents and families will acquaint them with programs, activities, staff, other residents and physical space.
2. Helping residents make choices and take responsibilities in order to maintain as much control as possible over their own lives.
3. Helping the resident to cope with losses associated with leaving the prior living situation.
4. Advocacy role for resident.
5. Continue maintaining family relationships and support for clear expectations of family's involvement.
6. Maintaining access to the community by working with individuals, organizations, and groups who have had past involvement with the resident.
7. Helping to create a personalized and supportive environment.

8. Assisting the resident to establish a life-style adapted to the nursing home. Resident develops roles and relationships, and participates in activities consistent with previous life-styles. Staff is encouraged to adapt nursing home routines to meet individual needs.
9. Helping the resident find meaning and purpose in his life in the nursing home consistent with previous values and goals. This is when adaptation and adjustment to the nursing home takes place.

Assessing and Planning Resident Care

The social worker collaborates with other members of the interdisciplinary team to plan care. From the social history, an assessment of psychosocial functioning is made. This information helps staff understand adaptive and maladaptive behaviors in a historical perspective, identify social and emotional needs, coping abilities, and resources. Psychosocial goals and approaches to enhance overall functioning are identified. The social worker may contribute to specific social service goals (e.g., need for financial assistance) involve problems related to other departments (i.e. lack of motivation to attend PT), or address goals of the total staff. The psychosocial assessment begins with a thorough history similar to the following:

1   **Background Information**
Birthdate   Cultural background
Birthplace   Religious affiliation and signifi-
Immigration date   cance
Education   Occupation and work history

2. **Family History and Relationship**
Marital status   Name and relationships of
Spouse's name   significant others
Date of marriage   Significant family events
Family (include children,   Family interactions (cohesion,
   grandchildren, siblings)   adaptations, communications)
   names and relationships   Family supports

3. **Social Functioning and Relationship; Social Networks**
Interpersonal relationships with significant others—past and present
Other social relationships, social skills, and communication patterns
Social activities
Community involvement, organization, activities
Support systems, resources

4. **Emotional Functioning/Mutual Functioning**
   Previous attitudes, feelings, behavioral pattern
   Changes in attitudes, feelings, behavioral pattern
   Observable behavior, coping pattern and adapting to change
   Mental status: memory, orientation, judgment, comprehension
   Self-concept: self-image, self-esteem

5. **Life-Style**
   Use of leisure time, interests, hobbies, recreational activities
   Daily habits—Likes, preferences, dislikes, idiosyncrasies
   Past life-style and significant life event
   Roles: past and present

6. **Medical History**
   Disability, functioning and adjustment to disability
   Perceptual functioning

7. **Admission to Nursing Home**

Previous living arrangement	Initial adjustment
Events leading to NH placement	Expectation and attitudes of both resident and family

The analysis and interpretation of this kind of data results in the identification of an individual's social and emotional problems, needs and strengths. From this, a goal oriented social service care plan is developed.

A social service care plan is written for all new patients as soon as possible after admission. It will be altered in the event of further losses or disability, specific cognitive or affective behaviors (especially depression or disruptive and self-destructive behaviors), a crisis situation, problems related to residents and staff, family problems, communication problems, chemical misuse, death and dying, relocation within the facility or discharge. Needs may include supportive equipment, specific services, financial assistance, and social or ego-related needs, e.g. need for acceptance or approval.

When working with the cognitively impaired resident, social services are adapted to meet the needs, capacities, and resources of that individual. Approaches must be appropriate for the resident's functional level. Nonverbal communication—touch, gestures, cues, and simplified verbal communications (frequent repetition and the use of simple explanations) are emphasized. The approaches must be consistent with the intervention techniques of other staff. Services for the severely impaired are apt to focus more on working with family and staff.

Ongoing Services

Advocacy/Resident Council

The social worker's function in resident advocacy is a crucial service to the resident and ultimately to the facility. It can best be provided by working with staff and not against staff and while all staff are advocates for the resident, the social worker will help to focus on this.

First, services are provided to assure patient rights. The social worker works with staff to assure such basic rights as human dignity and respect, as well as rights to confidentiality of information, individuality of care, and information regarding care and treatment. Residents have the right and the responsibility to make decisions regarding their care and treatment. The social worker helps staff and residents to work through these issues realistically. This may involve the resident in care planning, or the right to refuse care and treatment.

Residents have the right to be free from abuse. Abuse may come from other residents, friends, family, or staff. It may be legal, financial, verbal, or physical in form, or it may involve taking possessions or using undue restraints. Social services help to protect the resident by working with the resident and the persons involved.

Social services assist the resident to obtain services from family, community, and facility resources. When reasonable requests such as getting a pair of glasses or a psychological evaluation are denied, the social worker can become an advocate for the resident. Advocacy services also include listening and responding to resident complaints and the implementation of grievance procedures when appropriate.

Resident councils are an important vehicle for advocacy. They involve far more than making complaints and raising money. Resident councils can identify issues and problems and suggest actions to resolve them. The social worker can facilitate resident council suggestions.

Counseling/Crisis Intervention

Counseling may be an individual or group service for residents and families with coping, social, emotional, or behavioral problems. Basic to counseling is the quality of the relationship the worker has already established.

Counseling is a problem-solving and communication process. Carkhuff (1969) describes the components of a facilitative communication as: empathy, respect, genuineness, concreteness, selfdisclosure, and confrontation. These communication components are used in the counseling process. It is through the counseling process of verbalization, clarification, summarization, exploration of alternatives, and choosing a course of action, that the social worker helps residents develop coping skills and resolve problems addressed by the social service plan. Reassurance and education may also be part of the counseling process.

Crisis intervention differs from counseling. As implied, crisis intervention may be initiated when there is an immediate crisis such as "going on welfare," death of a resident, sudden illness, hospitalization, or decreased function. The objectives of crisis intervention are to reduce the impact of the stressful event and to utilize it to help the person solve the present problem and strengthen his coping abilities. During a crisis, even minimal therapeutic assistance can achieve the maximum benefit. In addition to verbalization and clarification, intervention employs the use of personal and institutional resources and sometimes modification of the environment. Counseling and crisis intervention skills are learned by the worker through training and experience.

Working With Families

On admission, the social worker helps the family to be immediately included in the life of the resident within the facility by sharing a meal or helping the resident settle in. The initial adjustment period is a time for concentration of social services because the family will soon be included or excluded from involvement with the resident in the home. Overall, social services to families include:

1. Assessment of family needs, family support, coping patterns, and family relationships.
2. Family orientation.
3. Family education—individually and in groups.
4. Information and referral to community resources.
5. Support and counseling—individually and in groups.
6. Family programming.
7. Involving families in resident care plans, approaches and care.

Special needs may arise such as physical or verbal abuse, overprotection, alienation or denial of a resident's illness or disabilities. In these cases the worker helps the family and resident develop more functional patterns of interaction through direct intervention or in consultation with other staff or community resources. The worker also assists families when there is a need for guardianship or financial assistance; and works closely with family during discharge planning.

Working With Groups

Group work adds an important dimension to social work services. Residents join together in a group which then develops an existence of its own. The interactions of group members and the group itself can help individual members to change and grow in ways that the social worker, working with individual residents, cannot.

Groups tend to be problem, change- or growth-oriented and focus on change within individuals or the group itself. In the former, a common problem is adjustment to a physical disability with individuals in the group bringing about change. Groups may address new residents, family support, loss and adjustment, sensory impairment, stroke, cancer groups, or socialization. The latter may be a common group living problem, such as smoking in the lounge. In this instance, it could be referred to the Resident's Council for a group solution.

Social group work uses a democratic process; decisions are made by members in a democratic manner, thus enhancing the resident locus of control. The leader is a facilitator, whose role will vary depending on the needs of the group and its ability to function.

Assisting With Relocation Within the Nursing Home

Residents may move from one room to another in the home because of a roommate problem, a desire for a different room, or a need to accommodate other residents. When residents are moved frequently and abruptly, the problem is identified as "apple cart upset."

When a move is contemplated, the social worker considers the resident's interest as primary. Is the move in the resident's best interest? What social and emotional factors are involved? Can interpersonal problems be resolved through counseling? Because the room is the resident's home, moving may create effects similar to those upon initial entry to the nursing home. In roles as advocate and case manager, the social worker considers alternative decisions and makes preparations that respect the resident's well-being.

Working With Dying Residents and Their Families

In the last stage of life, the social worker continues to address the psychosocial needs of both the dying resident and family. The social worker may help the resident talk about and work through reactions to his own death, help him review his life in order to understand its meanings and purposes, help to resolve conflicts, and assist him to plan and prepare for death. The worker also encourages close friends to listen and talk to the resident.

Family needs may become greater at this time. A family assessment includes their reactions, its effect on the family system and interaction with the resident. Support may include helping them express their feelings, providing information and helping them understand and support the dying person. Preparation for death also involves legal and financial preparations, planning the funeral, and disposing of possessions.

The worker collaborates with staff to create an environment that is supportive and responsive to the resident's total needs, calm but not isolating, and as reassuring as possible. The social worker continues to help the resident maintain control over decisions that affect him. In addition, other residents may need help in dealing with their reactions. Finally, both the social worker and staff will be affected and seek mutual support. Chapter 19 suggests many helpful ideas related to the subject of death and dying.

Discharge Planning

Discharge planning is a case manager function that provides continuity during transition within the health care system. It begins with preadmission assessment. The initial care plan includes a written discharge plan which is reviewed quarterly to assure appropriateness of placement. When there is little or no potential for discharge, planning is limited to goals for long-term placement. If a resident desires more independent living than his/her functional capacities support, the social worker can use the discharge assessment to counsel the resident. The worker reinforces realistic goals and attempts to help the resident decide on a more appropriate plan. When there is potential for more independent living or the resident seeks other living arrangements, discharge goals are then derived from assessment of:

Resident's motivation and goals for discharge
Resident's current level of functioning
Acceptable level of functioning for discharge
Need for supportive services, equipment and resources
Family motivation and goals regarding resident's discharge
Family support and services available
Available community support, services, and resources
Problems in discharge
Residents strengths and abilities for discharge
Alternative living situations

The social worker will coordinate services and resources with the nursing home staff, family, and community agencies and assist the resident and family with plans and preparations. Discharge assessment, plans, and activities are documented, and a discharge summary is written. Follow-up services are important to a successful discharge. It assures that the services and resources are being delivered as planned, that they are adequate, and that the resident is adjusting to the new living situation.

INDIRECT SERVICES IN THE FACILITY AND COMMUNITY

Modifying the Therapeutic Milieu

Residents living in a nursing home have been described as a "population at risk" by Gossett (1972). A consideration of the factors affecting morbidity and mortality rates of residents relocating to nursing homes support the view of this population being "at risk."

In order to address the total population, the total environment must be addressed. "A total therapeutic care approach . . . requires the examination of all actions, situations, policies, routines and programs for their effects upon the personal and social functioning of the resident population and the restructuring of these for therapeutic purposes," (Gossett, 1972). Many chapters of this book deal with these issues; staff roles, resident roles, adapting the physical environment, ways to humanize environments, change, managing the effects of institutionalization, and many administrative components.

The social worker supports goals to enhance staff to help residents become more functional—responsible, active and independent—rather than assuming the dysfunctional role of "patient." Together, staff help to create a supportive environment which is home-like and adaptive, flexible enough to meet resident's diversified needs and interests, stimulating as well as quieting. Staff encourages relationships between individual residents. The total effort can be enhanced by the social worker who can facilitate a therapeutic environment through realistic changes.

Collaborating and Coordinating With Community Resources

The nursing home will not be able to meet resident's needs in isolation from the community. Providing resources is a societal responsibility and a community endeavor. Therefore, the nursing home can best meet resident needs and supplement their own services by utilizing the community resources.

The social worker, as case manager, provides an interagency function by coordinating use of community resources and monitoring the activity with periodic assessment. The worker maintains a file of community resources for resident and family referral.

Referrals are made both to bring resources into the facility and to take residents out to the community. Referrals for financial assistance become a major responsibility of the social worker. Follow-up is again important to assure that the service was delivered and to evaluate the outcome.

Collaborating With Staff

Social services have an identifiable field of service in the nursing home, but these services often coincide with other disciplines. Nurses, for example, work with families, make referrals, provide social and emotional care, and implement a therapeutic milieu. Social workers do not make referrals to medical clinics, but they do to county social services. They do not regularly see all families, but they do see families with specific social or emotional needs or in family programs. Therefore, collaboration with other disciplines is essential.

Collaboration in care planning requires the contribution of each discipline for a holistic plan. It is important that staff discuss problems as they arise with residents and families in order to maintain open communication and respect for one another.

This is also true in the area of training and education. The worker's knowledge base and expertise can contribute to all caregivers. Education and training in the areas of social, emotional and behavioral functioning can be provided in staff orientation and inservice training formally. Informally, knowledge and insights can be shared through care conferences, social histories, charting, discussions with staff, and role-modeling with residents.

The social worker can also function as social worker for the staff by facilitating group interaction in meetings and conferences, and helping to open channels of communications and resolve conflicts. The worker can help staff cope with their own feelings regarding resident or family problems and provide information and referral for staff with personal problems. The social worker often becomes a supportive person for other staff.

Through membership on committees (utilization review, patient care, department head, etc.), the worker participates in determining policies or programs concerning the social and emotional aspects of care. Administrative support of sharing the expertise of all team members will enhance all services.

Documentation

Social services are responsible for documenting a social history and assessment of social and emotional health-related problems. It is updated when a resident is readmitted into the nursing home and when additional and valuable information has been gathered. A quarterly review of the psychosocial assessment is recommended to provide for any changes in the psychosocial needs of the resident.

A social service plan is written for all residents receiving social services, including residents participating in social service groups. This plan is a part of the overall plan of care and is a part of the medical record. It includes progress notes, a statement of the services provided, and an evaluation of goal achievement. It is also useful to maintain a file on residents with social service plans.

Social service policies and procedures must maintain confidentiality of documentation. Very sensitive information is not to be documented. Documentation should avoid the use of labels or diagnostic terms when no such diagnosis has been made—e.g., alcoholic, depression, paranoid.

SOCIAL WORK CONSULTATION

The purpose of social work consultation may be to design or assess the function of social services, provide case consultation, provide staff development, or other services. Consultation may function from outside the organization without authority or direct responsibility. The consultation process relies heavily on the use of problem-solving and education with the consultee (the facility). Recommendations for implementation are made to the administrator and to other staff directly involved in consultation. They may relate to any of the programs discussed throughout this chapter.

Sometimes, consultants function with direct responsibilities for implementing the social service program. In these situations the consultant may make assessments for resident care and write social service plans to be implemented by the worker. Implementation of the plan would be supervised by the consultant.

ADMINISTERING SOCIAL SERVICES

Administrative guidelines for social services are essential to the functioning of the department, the quality of services offered, and integration of services into the total organization. Though it may be a one-person department, it is important to have a clear mission statement and goals, policies and procedures, a job description, a budget, clear lines of responsibility to administration, and liaison with other departments. Social services need an office where interviews with residents and families can be conducted in private. Solid support from administration is essential for conducting an effective and quality social service program.

It is important for the social worker to consistently upgrade information, knowledge and skills in areas of long-term care, aging, social work and management. New knowledge and practices in long-term care and social work are continuous. As a worker gains experience, new knowledge and skill must be introduced into the services offered to maintain quality.

The administrator is responsible for selecting a social worker who is competent to provide the services described and evaluating the worker's performance and program. The administrator may consider the following criteria for hiring a social worker:

1. Training in the field of social work—preferably from an accredited school of social work.

2. Knowledge and skills basic to the social work profession and particularly to the services offered in the facility—skills in relationship building, verbal and written communication, assessment, admission and discharge planning, care planning, problem-solving, advocacy, counseling, group work, case management, linking formal and informal supports, aging, and long-term care.
3. Personal qualifications—a person who can communicate and relate positively to residents, families, and staff; who is accepting of others, warm and caring; assertive and a good advocate for residents, but also supportive of staff and administration; manages time well, takes initiative as part of a team; and maintains an ethical approach to social work.

SUMMARY

Social services make a unique contribution in the long-term care setting. They complement the predominantly medical and physical services by bringing the social and emotional component of care. They include direct services to residents and families and indirect services in collaboration with staff and community. While a full range of possible social services has been discussed, each facility must evaluate the needs of its residents and families, the organization's mission and goals, and facility and community resources in order to determine the components of its own social service department.

RECOMMENDED READINGS

Hooyman, Nancy and Nancy Lustbader. *Taking Care, Supporting Older People and Their Families,* New York, Macmillan Free Press, 1986.
Hottman, Elizabeth, *Social Services for the Elderly,* New York, Macmillan Co, 1985.
Silverstone, Barbara and A. Burack-Weiss. *Social Work Practice With the Frail Elderly and Their Families,* Springfield, IL, Charles C Thomas, 1983.

SUGGESTED READINGS

Bourestrom, N., and Tars, S. Alterations in life patterns following nursing home relocation. *Gerontologist, 13(6):*506–10, December 1974.
——————, Pastalan L: *Forced Relocation: Setting, Staff, and Patient Effects, Final Report.* Ann Arbor, Institute of Gerontology, University of Michigan, April, 1975.

Brieland, D. Definition, specialization and domain in social work. *Social Work, 26(1):*79–83, Jan., 1981.

Brody, E. The aging of the family. *Annals of the American Academy of Political and Social Science, 438(4):*13–27, July 1978.

Carkhuff, R. *Helping and Human Relations: A Primer for Lay and Professional Helpers. Selection and Training.* Vol. I. New York, Holt, Rinehart and Winston, Inc., 202–13, 1969.

—————. *Helping and Human Relations: A Primer for Lay and Professional Helpers. Practice and Research.* Vol. II. New York, Holt, Rinehart and Winston, Inc., 1969.

Coulton, C. Person-environment fit as the focus in health care. *Social Work, 26(1):*26–35, Jan. 1981.

Gossett, H. *A Curriculum for Social Work Personnel in Long-Term Health Care Facilities.* New York, National Association of Social Workers, Inc., 1972.

Lieberman, M. Relocation research and social policy. *The Gerontologist, 13( ):*494–501, Dec. 1974.

Minahan, A., and Pincus, A. A conceptual framework for social work practice. *Social Work, 22*(5):347–52, Sept. 1977.

Monk, A. Social work with the aged: principles and practice. *Social Work, 26*(1):61–8, Jan. 1981.

National Association of Social Workers. *Code of Ethics of the National Association of Social Workers.* Washington D.C., National Association of Social Workers, Inc., 1980.

National Association of Social Workers. *Standards for Social Work Services in Long-Term Care Facilities.* NASW Policy Statement No. 9, Washington D.C., National Association of Social Workers, Inc., 1981.

Pablo, R. Intra-institution relocation: its impact on long-term care patients. *The Gerontologist, 17*(5):426–34, Oct. 1977.

Chapter 17

ACTIVITIES: LIFE MEANS LIVING

JUDY EGGLESTON AND RUTH HASTINGS

INTRODUCTION

The long-term care facility has an obligation to provide rehabilitative care and life enrichment related to interpersonal relationships, maintenance of social roles, self-esteem and independence. In spite of individual limitations, residents have the right to the highest possible level of independence and meaning to their lives. If the organizational environment promotes meaningful living, there must be dynamic administrative leadership, an interdisciplinary team approach to resident care, maximum involvement of the resident in his or her daily life, and an effective activities department.

Activities programs can contribute to life enrichment in a way that no other program can. The goal is to provide opportunities for each resident to use existing abilities, build on past experiences, and to identify the motivations that will help each person to continue life's tasks. Individual and group programs consider limitations of participants but attempt to enhance each person's optimal level of functioning. They are not intended to correct a pathology or disability like a specialized rehabilitation service such as physical or occupational therapy, but they aim to prevent depression, promote greater self-esteem, and provide opportunities for positive social experiences.

When dependencies and frailities increase, individuals in nursing homes may require assistance in using their abilities to sustain their interests and involvement in living. Non-involvement leads to rapid mental, social and physical deterioration.

To meet the growing needs of nursing home residents, activities departments must expand their scope of programming. In addition, administrators, staff, volunteers, families and residents themselves must raise their expectations for resident outcomes. Low expectations are the single-most limiting factor in establishing creative and dynamic activities programs. If professionals in the field reflect society's attitudes and false perceptions of the elderly's capabilities, nursing home residents will not be given life enriching opportunities.

Appropriately selected activities give purpose to daily existence and stimulate the individual to use his/her existing capabilities as much as possible. It is through a well-designed activities program, more than anything else, that a resident is able to establish identity, maintain vital links with the community and live a meaningful life.

ACTIVITIES COORDINATOR—ROLE AND FUNCTION

An effective activities program responds to the older person's ability to learn, develop and adjust to new life situations and social roles. It is obligated to include as many forms of activity and self-expression as are normally pursued by all persons. In order to design and implement a creative and balanced program, an individual with specialized skills, knowledge, training and education is necessary to head the activities department. Experienced people are invaluable in implementing an activities program; however, education and training in health care, gerontology, administration and supervision, resident assessment, documentation and recordkeeping, group work and activity analysis are some components basic to the position of Activities Coordinator.

An Activities Coordinator is a full-time department head and a member of the professional staff. This individual is directly responsible to the facility's administrator or director of resident services, depending upon the organizational structure.

The Activities Coordinator should not be the person responsible for special facility events such as employee recognition/parties, National Nursing Home Week or the facility newsletter. These are best accomplished by facility committees to share in these responsibilities. Resident services such as personal shopping and appointments should also be shared by facility staff, family members and volunteers. The Activities Coordinator's primary responsibility is the coordination of resident activity.

The Activities Coordinator has both administrative and resident care responsibilities. Administrative management functions include, but are not limited to, the following:

1. Supervising staff and volunteers assigned to the activities department.
2. Recruiting, hiring and terminating activities personnel in conjunction with the administrator.
3. Orienting, annually evaluating and coordinating inservice education for activities personnel.
4. Developing and updating departmental policies, procedures and job descriptions.
5. Assessing and utilizing the resources within the facility and the community.
6. Providing orientation to the activities program for all new employees of the nursing home.
7. Providing inservice education for all nursing home staff in areas such as the therapeutic value of activities and therapeutic approaches that promote resident participation and social interaction.
8. Preparing the annual departmental budget and operating within its parameters.
9. Procuring and maintaining departmental supplies and equipment.
10. Preparing an annual report to administration and establishing goals and objectives for the coming year.
11. Evaluating the program to determine its effectiveness in meeting resident needs.

Resident care responsibilities include, but are not limited to, the following functions:

1. Obtaining an activity history and assessing the needs and interests of residents for activity.
2. Participating in or supervising the activities staff involvement in the care planning process.
3. Planning, scheduling and coordinating individual and group activities appropriate to the needs and interests of the residents and consistent with the individual's plan of care.
4. Documenting and evaluating each resident's participation in activities.

The intent of the activities program is to provide opportunities for all residents to engage in meaningful use of their time. The success of the activities program will depend upon the Activities Coordinator's ability to identify which things the residents are likely to choose to do and provide a way for the residents to do them. Too often the education, experience and abilities needed are underestimated. The ability to manage a department and plan and direct an activities program necessitates an individual with education, training, experience and a personality to perform the functions, along with the leadership of an enlightened administrator.

STAFFING

The number of staff and the staffing pattern of an activities department determine the amount of programming possible. A "9 to 5," five-day-per-week model cannot accommodate the variety of activities and programming needed. An activities program which encompasses a seven-day-per-week design, including late afternoon and evening activities, permits residents to pursue activity patterns of their previous lifestyle.

Weekend and evening activities can be accomplished through flexible hours of the activities staff or with other staff or volunteers being responsible for implementing programming coordinated by the activities department. Innovative programming depends on the flexibility, commitment and cooperation of the entire staff of the facility. Again, the achievement of this team effort is dependent upon the leadership of the facility's administrator.

The activities staff should include individuals with skills, talents and abilities that extend the opportunities available to the residents. The program can be further expanded by utilizing the talents and skills of other nursing home staff, family members and volunteers. A consultant can be used where the employment of an individual with special skills and background is not possible. Occupational therapists, therapeutic recreation specialists, group social workers, music therapists or experts in the therapeutic use of art, dance, poetry, literature, drama, horticulture and pets are valuable resources.

The activities department is commonly concerned with utilizing volunteers whose involvement can significantly enrich and extend the activities program. The Activities Coordinator should not, however, be expected to administer the facility's volunteer program.

DEPARTMENTAL RESPONSIBILITIES

Resident Assessment

An activities program will succeed only when the activities offered are based on a comprehensive assessment of the residents for whom the program is designed. A new resident cannot simply be informed of the kinds of scheduled activities available and then asked whether or not he/she might want to participate in some of them. This process attempts to fit residents into an established program. In order to offer activities that will motivate a resident to participate, information about his/her past activity involvement is necessary. This information will indicate the need to create new activities in response to a particular resident's needs and interests.

The Activities Coordinator obtains a comprehensive activity history on each resident. This history includes information about interests, abilities, special talents, ethnic background, educational and vocational experience, religious orientation, family system, pattern of social interaction and use of leisure time. It is important to create a picture of how the resident has spent his/her time. What was the pattern of sleep, rest and activity? What was the frequency and duration involved in particular tasks and in what setting? How many other people were involved? What areas of interest has the resident wanted to pursue but never had the opportunity to experience? As much as possible, this information should be obtained directly from the resident. If needed, the family and friends also provide useful information.

The resident's functional status is assessed by the Activities Coordinator and other professionals to determine the extent to which the resident's disability and specific behaviors may interfere with participation in activities. These areas include mobility, self-care, sensory and physical impairments, communication, orientation, cognition and behavior. This information is essential to the development of a **realistic** individualized activities plan.

Individualized Activities Plans

An individualized activities plan is developed for each resident. This plan is part of the resident care plan which is developed by an interdisciplinary team, the resident and the family. The resident care plan is based on each service's assessment of the resident. Individual resident needs are identified and interdisciplinary goals are established to coordinate and integrate staff and resident efforts.

The individualized activities plan is based on the **problems** or **needs** of the resident, interdisciplinary resident goals established at the care conference, and any precautions and limitations identified by the physician or other health care professionals. The activities **approach** to meet the identified needs of the resident is determined by activity history, preferences and functional ability of the resident, the organized facility activities program, and the available facility and community resources. This plan must be available to all activities staff, and it must be reviewed and revised as changes occur. The plan should, at all times, reflect what the activities department is providing for the resident. The resident's response is recorded in progress notes on the resident's chart.

Activities Program

The activities offered depend upon the capabilities and interests of the residents and the available facility and community resources. Regardless of the reason for admission, most long-term care residents experience difficulties with interpersonal relationships, social withdrawal, isolation and lack of self confidence. However, the causative factors are different for each individual. An activities program is made up of two components: 1) **an environment** that provides stimulation and creates opportunity for spontaneous interaction, and 2) a planned **program** of individual and group activities to meet the normal needs and interests of all residents in the facility.

Environment: A dynamic and motivating climate of participation is created by a home-like atmosphere, one that offers the residents as much as possible the kind and variety of choices they had in their own homes. The Activity Coordinator contributes much to the variety and choices available to the resident in managing his/her time. These spontaneous activities are not a part of the regularly scheduled programs. An environment filled with growing plants, aquariums, bird feeding stations, pets, thermometers by windows, seasonal decorations, selected **periodic** background music, news announcements, photographs, art exhibits, current magazines, puzzles, games and writing materials on desks will provide stimulation and create opportunity for spontaneous individual and small group interaction. This kind of environment depends upon the efforts and flexibility of all services/departments in the facility.

The scheduling of activities must respond to the normal sleep, rest and activity pattern of each resident. This is only possible when all schedules of daily care (such as baths and bedtimes) are coordinated with opportunities for activities at times that reflect the resident's previous lifestyle. Some people are accustomed to sleeping or napping in the afternoon and staying up late at night. Not everyone is ready for activity in the morning or sufficiently stimulated by mid-afternoon. Opportunities to engage in planned as well as spontaneous activities must be made available during the late afternoon and evening hours.

Weekend programs are essential. Many residents do not have visitors or go on family outings, a reason commonly given for the lack of weekend programs. Saturdays and Sundays are particularly lonely. There are fewer doctors' visits, special treatments and general facility business. A creative approach to staffing patterns and staff functions, community resources and utilization of volunteers will assist in finding a solution to this all too frequent problem.

Planned Program: A comprehensive activities program provides activities designated to respond to resident needs which can be categorized as follows: **physical, intellectual, social, creative, spiritual** and **emotional.** It is apparent that most activities respond to more than one need area to a greater or lesser degree. For example, gardening is generally thought of in terms of physical exercise. However, it also provides intellectual stimulation of growing plants, weather conditions and changing seasons; emotional satisfaction through caring for plants; and social interaction through recognition of results accomplished, and shared group tasks. All activities can be analyzed for the presence of these elements and adapted to different levels of resident function. Consideration is given to the components present in each activity which can be planned or implemented by the residents **themselves.** Too often, staff and volunteers do too much for the resident, denying them the opportunity to contribute. Residents will participate best in activities relevant to their particular needs, interests and abilities and that are the result of their own ideas and efforts.

Special attention needs to be given to the expressive arts of music, art, dance and literature; vehicles of personal expression and inspiration that have provided meaning and hope to persons in all circumstances of life through both the active, creative process as well as responsive role. Through the arts, persons can come to know their own unique contribution essential to positive self-esteem and be made aware of their common concerns shared with other persons. The expressive arts experience can be readily adapted to many levels of physical and psycho-social function as well as to various combinations of individual and group formats. Active self expression and awareness of personal uniqueness and a sense of community are the special therapeutic benefits of creative arts programs.

Intergenerational programs are also an essential component of an activities program. The nursing home provides a unique valuable resource for developing opportunities for sharing with children and young adults. In recent years with the increased awareness of issues on aging, most schools, churches, service clubs and community agencies are eager to become involved with nursing home residents. The wise administrator and Activities Coordinator will respond to these relationships with knowledge, skill and originality. Successful programs do require careful conception, planning and preparation of participants. However, the rewards are great not only in the obvious benefits of the present, but also as investments in the future. Young people who have good experiences with the elderly in nursing homes today will develop positive attitudes about aging and nursing homes.

A comprehensive activities program includes opportunities to engage in a wide variety of normal social relationships, which range from being alone to large assembly type activities. There are many daily tasks that are normally done **alone** such as reading, writing letters, watching TV, listening to records, or sewing. Most people look forward to some period of privacy each day to review their thoughts, pray or simply do nothing. This is particularly difficult in a nursing home setting. One way to provide more privacy is to encourage roommates to participate in activities at different times, allowing each individual some time to be alone in his/her room.

In the normal course of daily activity, much time is spent in activities with one to six persons, such as visiting, mealtime, games and walking. These activities are routine or spontaneous. Participation in groups of this size is most likely to elicit social interaction and promote enduring friendships. Little time is normally spent in large group activities which usually require more planning and effort. These include church services, sporting events, movies, plays and concerts. Large group activities can be very stimulating but they often do not involve active participation or **require** social interaction.

Traditional emphasis in activities programming is placed on the extreme end of the continuum; large spectator assemblies and efforts for one to one visits. These extremes are not supportive of enduring, meaningful social relationships. Smaller group activities offered are less well defined and organized. This is unfortunate since ongoing involvement in special need or interest groups provide the resident with a sense of belonging which has often been disrupted by relocation from familiar surroundings.

The social interaction resulting from carefully designed group involvement has a proven potential for motivating residents to learn new, meaningful life roles in a congregate institutional setting. Planning is essential. A group **purpose** must be established and group membership must be selective. The types of groups developed depend upon the assessed needs and interests of the residents and the resources available in the facility and community. Five kinds of ongoing group programs particularly appropriate for long-term care facilities are:

1. Orientation for new residents and their families (see Chapters 16 and 19).
2. Special interest groups in order to share common experiences, pursue past hobbies, or learn new skills.
3. Special need groups in order to assist residents with common problems or needs (e.g., stroke, arthritis, overweight, cognitive disorders).
4. Resident government to provide opportunities to be involved in decisions that affect their daily life in the facility.
5. Community relations to provide opportunities to participate in the life of the community and to host community members in the facility.

It is social interaction more than anything else that determines the success of a person's ability to cope with the losses of aging and disability. Satisfying social interaction and a sense of belonging enable a person to maintain his/her identity, develop new life roles and establish new ways of being.

Therapeutic Approaches

Some residents are unable to engage in satisfying social interaction. Common reasons for this in the elderly are disorientation, memory loss, depression, isolation and sensory deprivation. Therapeutic techniques designed to promote social interaction and functional independence can be classified into four general categories: orientation to reality, motivation, sensory stimulation and active listening (Figure 17-1). Many programs

Figure 17-1

THERAPEUTIC APPROACHES THAT PROMOTE SOCIAL INTERACTION

	Orientation to Reality	*Motivation*	*Sensory Stimulation*	*Active Listening*
Resident Problem	disoriented to time, place or person	inactive, withdrawn unmotivated apathetic not involved with others	diminished sensory perceptions; i.e. vision and hearing impairments; isolated and inactive	depressed, angry acting out behaviors, withdrawn, isolated.
Resident Goal	oriented to time, place and/or person	to motivate to social or task involvement; to interact with the environment	to strengthen sensory perception and increase meaningful contacts with the environment	to work through depression; accept self and circumstances
Staff Action	provide repetition and consistency of information about person, place and time.	provide positive emotional stimulation through recalling past events; experiences and personal accomplishments	provide varied sensory stimuli for all 5 senses through environmental adaptation and special activities	provide opportunity to *identify and express feelings* about past and/or present events or circumstances in their life
Representative Activities	current events exercises gardening familiar games music sing-along special luncheons weather reports bird-watching time-lines	autobiography baking cards gardening community visits remotivation poems/stories/ Rockwell prints holiday celebration music pets family parties	Balloon volleyball blow bubbles baking dancing exercise gardening music sing-alongs tasting parties pets	companion program discussion groups pastoral visits life review time-lines

and activities become a combination of these and can also be adapted for one-on-one experiences.

It is important to emphasize that these approaches are designed to deal with specific problems and needs. Which approach will benefit which resident is a determination of the care planning team. Successful results depend upon consistent application by all staff, volunteers and family members. For example, the nursing staff can focus on orientation information while giving daily care, the dietary staff during mealtime, and the family members or volunteers during visits or on outings. Effective utilization of these approaches depends upon a staff that is trained in their use and knows when to use them.

FACILITY RESOURCES

Physical Plant

Too many long-term care facilities have been designed without activities in mind. Much work is being done to design environments that will promote resident involvement in a much greater variety of activities. Space on each living unit convenient to resident rooms greatly facilitates resident participation. The fact remains, however, that programs must be developed within the limits of existing resources. One thing is clear, spaces allocated for activities must be flexible and multi-purpose, and staff must view the entire facility for creative uses.

There needs to be space available for:

- assembly size groups
- small group meetings; some of which offer privacy
- individual activities
- quiet, clean activities
- noisy activities
- active games
- messy activities
- cooking facilities
- outdoor areas, including garden space and walking paths with appropriate benches, handrails and shade

Space and equipment needed at any given time will change with the needs of the residents. The list of possible activities that might benefit the residents is limited only by the imagination of the program planners.

Transportation

Transportation is a requirement for many common everyday activities such as shopping, visits to community events, dining out and sightseeing. This must be provided by the facility or arrangements made with outside resources. Insurance policies need to be reviewed to give adequate protection for driver and passengers. Drivers must be oriented to the general needs of the residents and staff or volunteers must be available to provide assistance to residents with special needs. No activities program can function successfully without some means of transportation readily available.

Budget

The operational plan for financing activities is usually a projection of financial requirements for one year. Budget planning must include:

1. Staff salaries
2. Permanent equipment—purchase, maintenance and repair
3. Expendable supplies
4. Special projects or events
5. Overhead
6. Transportation
7. Professional development/continuing education

Activities should not be supported by monies generated from the sale of craft items. It may be very beneficial to the residents to earn money through their efforts; however, their involvement must be clearly voluntary. The decision concerning the use of such funds must be left up to the residents through some mechanism as the Resident Council. Examples of the uses of these funds might include purchasing of equipment needed to augment the activities program in the facility (e.g., VCR, large screen TV). Other uses may be contributing the funds to a community service agency or project, or using the funds for a special event for the residents who participated in the task (e.g., attend a cultural event or ball game). Policies and procedures need to be developed in regard to any profit-making activities, whether for an individual resident or for the facility at large.

COMMUNITY RESOURCES

Every effort must be made to utilize all available community resources in order to provide the resident's continued involvement in the community consistent with his/her previous lifestyle and to expand and enrich the activities program. Opportunities must exist for the residents to participate in the community as well as for the residents to host community activities and events. Every community offers different possibilities and which ones will benefit the most residents depends upon the particular needs of the residents and the facility. However, **every** organization, agency and institution in the community must be scrutinized for the possibilities they may offer the nursing home and visa versa. A list of community resources includes:

- Schools
- Adult Education Programs
- Church
- Libraries
- Museums
- Historical Societies
- State/Municipal Arts
- Councils
- Day Care Centers
- Boy & Girl Scouts
- 4-H Clubs
- YWCA/YMCA
- Theaters/Drama Groups
- Orchestras/Bands/Choirs
- Service Organizations
- Zoos
- Shopping Centers
- Local Industries & Businesses
- Hobby Groups
- Political Action Groups
- Nature Clubs
- Resorts
- Farms
- Self-Help Organizations
- Newspaper/Radio/TV Stations

The role of the Activities Coordinator is to orient the resource person to the needs and abilities of the residents, to the facility and to assess residents for potential involvement. He/she must view herself as a **coordinator** in the true sense of the word and utilize the expertise available.

SUMMARY

It is apparent that the administrator plays a crucial role in influencing the quality of the activities program. He/she must be committed to the inherent value of the program as it relates to the health and life satisfaction of residents. The activities department is an integral part of resident care and cannot accomplish its purpose without communication and coordination with all other resident care services. This team approach depends upon the leadership of the administrator.

Creative and responsive activities programming requires a heavy investment in staff development and a willingness to try innovative ways of utilizing facility and community resources. An adventurous attitude will result in the exploration of new kinds of resident and staff experiences consistent with the positive expectation of what can be accomplished through careful planning and facility-wide support. In spite of the uncertainties sometimes present in untried activities, the administrator must be willing to take a chance and assume the challenge.

Vigorous, systematic efforts must be directed toward the assessment of functional ability and capacity for adaptive living. Reticence in trying this positive approach is mainly due to the low expectations and false perceptions of aging and disability held by society and to the persistence of a hospital model which emphasizes sickness and disabilities. The focus must be shifted to **ability** and capacity for adaptive living.

The preventable disabilities are those that result from disuse. Providing opportunities to exercise all existing abilities on a regular basis in ways that are meaningful to the resident is the challenge and responsibility of all departments. The process begins by assessing each resident for all tasks that he/she can do and for the kinds of activities he/she is most likely to choose.

Activities offered must require the active involvement of the resident as much as possible while providing whatever assistance is necessary. This balance between maximum resident involvement in the selection and planning, as well as participation, and the amount and kind of assistance provided is central to the therapeutic benefits of the activity. Because the need for activity is daily, activities must be scheduled for seven days a week and include late afternoon and evening hours. This will require flexible staffing schedules, interdepartmental cooperation and the use of outside resources.

Satisfying social interaction is a strong motivating factor for the maintenance of health in long-term care. This is best accomplished through activities designed in small group settings that can promote the development of enduring friendships and new life roles and purposes. The traditional emphasis on large assembly type activities and one to one resident and staff encounters must be expanded to include a dynamic variety of small group programs.

The administrator's responsibility is to 1) support the activities program with a mission statement and philosophy upon which it can build; 2) select a well qualified Activities Coordinator; 3) provide an environment that encourages varied and innovative activities and promotes mastery; 4) provide financial resources for the program; and 5) evaluate the outcomes of the program in terms of life satisfaction of the residents.

REFERENCES AND RESOURCES

Breuer, J. *A Handbook of Assistive Devices for the Handicapped Aged.* New York, Haworth Press, 1982.

Killeffer, E.H.P et al, Ed. *Handbook of Innovative Programs for the Impaired Elderly.* New York, Haworth Press, 1984.

Peterson, C. and S. Gunn. *Therapeutic Recreation Program Design,* Englewood Cliffs, NJ, Prentice-Hall, 1984.

Teaff, J. *Leisure Services with the Elderly,* St. Louis, Times Mirror/Mosby, 1985.

Tiara, D., Ed. *Physical and Occupational Therapy in Geriatrics,* New York, Haworth Press, 1984.

Weiss, Caroline and Judi Kronberg. "Upgrading TR Service to Severely Disoriented Elderly," *Therapeutic Recreation Journal,* First Quarter, 1986.

Zgola, Jitka M. *Doing Things. A Guide to Programing Activities for Persons with Alzheimer's Disease and Related Disorders,* Baltimore, MD, Johns Hopkins University Press, 1986.

ORGANIZATIONAL RESOURCES

American Art Therapy Association, Inc.
Business Office
428 East Preston Street
Baltimore, MD 21202

The American Dance Therapy Association, Inc.
2000 Century Plaza, Suite 230
Columbia, MD 21044

American Library Association, Inc.
Association of Specialized and Cooperative Agencies
50 E. Huron Street
Chicago, IL 60611

American Occupational Therapy Association
1383 Piccard Drive
Rockville, MD 20850.

American Theater Association, Inc.
1000 Vermont Avenue, N.W.
Washington, DC 20005

National Association of Activity Professionals
520 Stewart
Park Ridge, IL 60068

The National Association for Music Therapy, Inc.
P.O. Box 610
Lawrence, KS 66044

The National Educational Council of Creative Therapies, Inc.
20 Rip Road
Hanover, NH 03755

National Recreation and Park Association
3101 Park Center Drive
Alexandria, VI 22302

Chapter 18

ENVIRONMENTAL ADAPTATIONS TO COMPENSATE FOR SENSORY CHANGES

MARGARET CHRISTENSON

Introduction

The relationship of the physical environment to dependencies of residents is one of the most overlooked areas of patient care. Because the research in this area is often unknown to administrators who must plan that environment, it is essential for them to understand the areas in which their influence can improve both physical and mental functioning.

As people age, certain sensory changes cause them to become more dependent on the environment for support. While the age of onset and the rate of decline differ markedly among and within the various sensory systems, changes are gradual and most people are able to function adequately at home and in familiar surroundings. This so-called sensory deprivation is of course greater in the institutionalized elderly.

Obviously, losses in more than one sense increases a person's overall problems. Parent has summarized the effects of sensory deprivation which include: the loss of the ability to concentrate, disorientation and reported hallucinations, and delusions.

It is also thought that human interaction with the environment and its objects has a major role in eliciting intelligent behavior. Many researchers contend that coping with appropriate environmental complexity contributes to mental function. Lawton has studied environments on the basis of their behavioral demands. Varying degrees of "environmental press" can challenge the more competent individual or cause maladaptive behavior for those with multiple losses.

This chapter deals with age-related changes in vision, hearing, taste, smell, touch and kinesthetic systems, and whenever possible, suggests environmental modifications that can compensate for the changes in each of these systems. The administrator's task is to make the physical environment as supportive to physical and mental functioning of residents as possible. This does not mean that the administrator must be technically expert at interior design and decoration. It does, however, mean that the administrator must be attuned to the issues, know where the resources are, and be a role model for staff, families, and consultants. The administrator must demonstrate commitment to developing a supportive physical environment and encouraging others to do the same.

Visual Adaptations

In a study of 295 extended care residents by Snyder, 24 percent were legally blind (20/200 with correction), and 35 percent had low vision (20/70 to 20/100 with correction). This may be typical of many homes, but each home must screen all new residents and all residents annually to know the extent of visual problems in a particular facility and to determine changes in individual residents.

Visual Aids

Large contrasting lettering on signs and on written directions will facilitate vision for the person with acuity problems. Letters for signs should be a minimum of ⅝ inch in height and preferably recessed or raised 1/32 inch for readability through touch. Whether letters should be light colored on a dark colored background or dark letters on a light colored background depends on the visual problem and the lighting. In any case, lettering on signs must contrast markedly with the background (Sicurella). Name tags for staff should have large lettering. A largeprint calendar in a corridor can function both as landmark and an orienting aid.

Many items useful to low-vision persons are available through the American Foundation for the Blind. These devices include specially adapted watches and clocks. The partially sighted can benefit from self-care techniques used by the blind; for example, leaving in place commonly used items and arranging food and utensils in the same places. From the Library of Congress, books and periodicals with larger print are available to allow the older person to continue reading.

Lighting. As the lens of the eye becomes less transparent and thickens and the pupil becomes smaller, an increased amount of light is required. Reading and close work can be aided by increased illumination. The 20-year-old uses a 100-watt bulb for visual tasks, the 40-year-old requires 145 watts; the 60-year-old 230 watts; and the 80-year-old 415 watts.

(Cristarella) However, bulbs should not be exposed or directly in the resident's line of vision since this creates direct glare.

Glare may develop from either a direct or indirect source. Direct glare occurs when light reaches the eye directly from its source. Indirect glare arises when the light reflects into the eye rebounding off of another surface. Sunlight shining on a highly polished floor is intolerable to the aging eye. Light is intensified as it is reflected off chrome wheelchairs, walkers, plastic-covered furniture, and waxed floors. Even dishes and silverware can reflect more light than is comfortable.

There are several ways of eliminating indirect glare. Avoid using glossy paint and shiny laminated plastic table tops. Windows may be covered with glare reducing film, tinted mylar shades, mini-blinds or pleated polyester window shades. The dull rather than the shiny side of poster board should be used to make signs and posters. Lobby directions and other glass-covered surfaces should have non-glare glass.

Outdoor seating areas should be provided with sun screens. Gazebos, wood trellises and fences have been used. Roof overhangs, awnings, or building recesses could limit direct sunlight penetration. To reduce glare, the location and type of trees should be studied to shade court-yards and major glass areas.

Wall-mounted valance or cove lighting that conceals the source of light, spreads it indirectly upon the ceiling and down on the floor to eliminate glare. Better lighting will make it easier for older persons to recognize faces and improve communications. A study by Snyder (1976) showed that increased accidents in a nursing home seemed to be directly related to energy conservationists who turned out every other light in the hall, causing the contrast between bright and shadowed areas of the hallways to appear as steps, particularly to people with perceptual difficulties.

Fluorescent fixtures can reduce glare, but they must be selected carefully and ballasts need to be checked to be sure flickering is minimized. "Fluorescent light flicker which eludes many younger persons is quite evident to older people, causing tearing, headaches and general inattentiveness. Exposed lamp fixtures and improperly functioning ballasts may be causes" (Hiatt, 1979). Fluorescent lighting should be combined with incandescent lighting in specific areas of maximum light usage, e.g., bathrooms, reading areas, and so on. Whenever fluorescent light sources are used, choose warm-white deluxe or prime color tubes. Parabo-loid patterned fixture covers on fluorescent lights, which are made of anodized aluminum and often used in libraries, provide better light distribution.

Fluorescent lighting has been eliminated from some "senile dementia units" because of the flickering that can occur. (Peppard) The inattentiveness that has been observed in the general older population due to flickering, may impact on the agitation that is a part of the behavior observed in the senile dementia population.

Some government rules and regulations run counter to what researchers have found about the aging process. Many states, for example, require ceiling lights in the middle of each room in a nursing home. When lying down, these lights create direct glare.

Exterior lighting should be evaluated. Post fixtures which are placed at eye level cause direct glare and should not be used. Better lighting is produced with covered lighting, 18 to 24 inches from the ground, which lights the ground surface evenly.

In an older person, sight recovery is delayed when moving from a light to a darker area. For example, coming from the outside on a sunny day into a dimly lit hallway it is more difficult for the older person to adapt. Moving into a much lighter area also creates problems. For an older person, turning on a light in a dark room can produce the same effect that one experiences when a flashbulb flashes (Hatton). When older persons must come from a light area to a darker area, such as into a foyer or into their own room from a hall, no furniture or other objects should be placed by the door. Residents need time for sight recovery. In addition, night lights should be installed in and on the way to the bathroom. A switch on the outside of the bathroom, with a light built into the switch plate as a night aid, can be very helpful.

Color Perception. With increasing age the lens of the eye takes on a yellowish color which impairs the perception of certain colors, particularly greens, blues, and purples. Dark shades of navy, brown, and black are probably not distinguishable except under the most intense lighting conditions. Pastel colors such as blues, beiges, yellows and pinks are often impossible to distinguish.

One study indicated a preference on the part of older persons for primary, secondary, or tertiary colors rather than pale pastels. Color schemes can make use of both cool and warm color ranges. One is not limited to red, orange, yellow, or rose. Blue and green tones can be just as effective. The goal for color when designing for the elderly is to not only make an area more aesthetically pleasing, but to help contrast different areas or an object from its background.

Since colors appear different according to the surface texture and the amount of light, they must be selected in conjunction with these considerations. When beige, pastel yellow, and pale green are used without the addition of texture on walls, for bedspreads, or for the cubicle curtains, there may be little differentiation.

Sicurella writes "even the complete absence of glare and the most appropriate lighting, though unquestionably necessary, may do little to help visually impaired persons to see an object if there is insufficient color contrast." When a jigsaw puzzle is available for residents, care should be taken that the table surface contrasts well with the puzzle pieces. The use of color and/or texture differences can clarify boundaries. The color of the wall and floor should contrast and carpet should not be run up the wall.

Creating a beneficial psychological response through the use of color is a controversial topic. Studies have been reported that certain responses can elicit certain behavior. The reaction to a color is based on our cultural background, lighting, texture, and other less obvious interactions. "We cannot arbitrarily say that a color will produce a given effect in behavior of all patients until research accounts for the interactive effect of all these variables" (Hiatt, 1985).

Color Coding. Color coding should be striking. One must also be aware of pattern, when dealing with color coding. Large graphic patterns for orientation have little cultural meaning for the older person. They may even create an institutional feeling. Different styles of furniture, combined with a particular picture or wall hanging give cues of a certain floor or area and may be more aesthetically acceptable. Familiar cultural cues, i.e., barber pole by a barber shop, are helpful.

Color coding can provide clear cues for orientation as well as break the monotony of long halls and large spaces. In a study done by Liebowitz at the Weiss Institute in Philadelphia, contrasting colors occurred frequently as accents in door jambs, nursing stations, graphics and room decor. Cooper used color cuing to demonstrate the favorable effect of enriching the environment with specific placement of color and light.

Reducing the amount of information in a corridor can also be facilitated through the use of color. Doorways that have no function for the residents, e.g., storage, linen room, locker rooms, etc. may be painted the background color of the walls. Ultimately, color cuing for directional purposes may not be as effective as object cues. The shape of an object, unusual architecture, a large plant, a window with a view, etc. as well as smells, air currents, and tactile cues all give the older person input as to place. Color is simply one of many ways we have of differentiating places, and it should be used in conjunction with texture, shapes and lighting (Cristarella, Hiatt, 1979).

Depth Perception. Depth perception depends on brightness and contrast, so any age-related process that affects the amount of light reaching the retina also affects depth perception. Many studies use tests emphasizing figure-ground perceptions.

These illusions are perceptual fluctuations in which an object or figure may suddenly be perceived as background and the background as a figure. The ability to recognize a simple visual figure when it is embedded in a complex figure background is also difficult. Studies suggest that it may be more difficult for an older individual to discern an object on a surface with an intense pattern background.

Figure-ground problems with the elderly have specific implications when selecting floor covering. As we age, we rely on color changes and contrasts (between light and dark colors) to signal changes in floor surfaces or steps or obstacles. Sometimes these detailed outlines or objects cannot be seen because of loss of depth perception. When pattern is present, as on a floor surface, it may appear to be an object or several objects. The avoidance of patterns on floor surfaces (including stripes, checks, and designs), particularly in hallways, lounges, or dining rooms, is strongly recommended (Hiatt, 1980).

Patterned floors pose particular difficulties for older people who are somewhat mentally confused. They may perceive patterns as objects but not be able to ask questions or identify the reality. This problem is observed when residents "step over" or reach for support on highly contrasting figured ground surfaces.

Other Considerations. In the environment of the person with senile dementia, what is **not** included visually is also an important consideration. To redirect the confused resident, doorways may be camouflaged with barriers or room dividers to disguise exits, doorhandles or call buttons (Hiatt, 1987). Since a confused resident will often follow others, care should be taken by staff and visitors how they enter and leave the unit (Schafer).

Eyeglasses may be a problem. Many institutionalized individuals are unable to clean their own glasses. The build-up of sticky fingerprints can result in visual alterations that render glasses virtually useless, so daily cleaning should be a part of nursing care. Bows need tightening every three to six months.

Atrophy of the muscles of the eyelid cause another visual problem. Studies that measured the upward and downward limit of gaze in the elderly found that the average upward gaze was 40 degrees for 5 to 14 year olds and 16 degrees for the 75 to 94 year olds. This research, combined with the low visual acuity of many residents and the fact that residents have an average height of 5 feet 5 inches and may be in wheelchairs requires special attention to the maximum height of landmarks and signs. When making any visual alterations in the environment, designers should place themselves at the resident's eye-level and take into account the visual limitations of the people for whom they are designing. Residents should be asked to test any planned alterations before final installations.

Steffens and Thralow found a significantly reduced visual field in the patients with Alzheimer's disease in comparison to the findings with the other demented patients. This gives additional credence to the lowered placement of signs and pictorial landmarks as well as the necessity of staff using these landmarks when attempting to orient residents.

Hearing Adaptations

Hearing loss may have an even greater psychological influence on a person than does the loss of vision. The feeling of "deadness" and depression from curtailed relationships often overwhelms both the suddenly deafened and those in whom deafness develops gradually. There is a strong correlation between hearing loss and depression. Indeed, the inability to distinguish words clearly can lead to rejection and withdrawal—either self-inflicted or imposed by others. In some instances, varying degrees of paranoia can be observed.

There are three kinds of hearing loss: conductive, central and sensorineural. They can occur alone or in combination. In conductive hearing loss, increasing the intensity (louder speech or mechanical amplification with a hearing aid) may permit the individual to hear. Auditory nerve centers within the brain are affected in a central hearing impairment. In the elderly, the most common source of auditory problems is a sensorineural loss known as presbycusis.

Presbycusis is caused by damage to the nerve endings and auditory hair cells in the inner ear. These combined losses result in difficulty in hearing high frequency sounds such as a high pitched voice or a shrill whistle. In addition, consonants carry less acoustic power than vowels. As a result, high frequency problems arise from the inability to discern certain consonants—for example: p, s, th, k, ha, s, sh, and ch. As a result, the older individual is unable to discriminate between phonetically similar words.

Brothen reported, "people may hear words as if they sat on top of each other." Instead of hearing, "How are you feeling today?"—the older person may hear, "howareyoufeelingtoday?" Waiting a second or two for the blurred message to be processed and repeating the information slowly and distinctly will make it easier for the person to understand what has been said (Bowersox). Rewording sentences also may be helpful when consonants are misunderstood.

Radio, television, and music in a nursing home need to be assessed carefully. If volume and treble are increased in relation to the bass, the listener is exposed to overload in the lower tones. Generally, persons with presbycusis are aided if the bass is turned up and the treble is turned down (Hiatt, 1979). Because of distortions, music in a high key serves to frustrate and distract rather than relax the person with presbycusis, and background music interferes with hearing daily conversations. Music groups that perform in the nursing home ideally should not use flutes and high soprano tones. Speakers and entertainers should be encouraged to use a microphone because this not only amplifies sound but also cuts out some high frequencies, making it easier for the person with presbycusis to hear. Sound amplification should be available on all telephones used by the hearing impaired.

Hearing Aids. Acceptance of hearing aids has increased dramatically in the last few years, mainly because of the improved cosmetic appearance. However, smaller hearing aids are a mixed blessing because they require fine hand and finger dexterity, sometimes beyond the physical capacities of older persons. Some older persons with presbycusis receive only partial benefits from a hearing aid because they often make the distortions louder.

Hearing screening should be done for all residents on admission and at least once a year. If a hearing aid is prescribed by an audiologist a trial period can be established to determine if the person will benefit from it. Some older persons may not use hearing aids because of old batteries, improper fit, lack of effectiveness, etc. When a resident needs assistance to insert the aid correctly, clean the earmold, or change the batteries, it must be included in the care plan.

Assistive listening devices may be used when hearing aids are not effective. They consist of a microphone and earphones and are not designed for continuous wear. The resident wears earphones and the microphone is placed close to the speaker or source of music. These devices may be obtained from an audiologist, local hearing association or stores that carry optical equipment.

Background Noise and Communication. Many elderly people with impaired hearing feel isolated because they are reluctant to eat in restaurants or attend large social gatherings because they cannot enjoy the conversation of people around them. In rooms where interaction is desired, background sound needs to be reduced. The sound from loud conversations, dishes, fans, television, traffic, music, etc., greatly interferes with hearing. Intercoms should be used as little as possible because the sound produces additional background interference and sometimes causes confusion. In dining rooms, persons with an identified hearing loss should not be placed near the kitchen or other noisy areas.

Moving into the field of vision and getting the person's attention before starting to speak are essential elements in communicating with the hearing impaired person. To facilitate lip reading, one should look directly at the person and speak slowly and distinctly. Shouting is not only unnecessary but causes mouth distortions that make lip reading difficult.

Persons with presbycusis require fire and smoke alarms (which usually have a high frequency sound) with a visual cue, such as a flashing light. The inability to identify a sound or to determine the source of a sound can create auditory illusions. For instance, one resident mistook the hum of her room air humidifier for a television set which she assumed the nurses had on all night. These illusions can be explored with the resident and the cause of the confusion explained.

Television and/or radio need to be controlled. Radios and television are ideally used to provide a focus for socialization and stimulation. A schedule of television preferences and use could be established by the residents' council.

It is important that the administrator and staff become sensitive to the problems created by overload of auditory sensory input. Snyder (1978) demonstrated that wandering and confusion increased in nursing homes during shift changes and other periods of high noise level. Hall reports that patients on an Alzheimer's unit that had minimum traffic, no television sets, no intercom or public address system, and no ringing phones showed reduced anxiety. In addition, no medications were passed at mealtime and residents ate in small groups, reducing noises that were related to the traditional dining room.

Acoustics. "Poorly managed and designed acoustical settings can be as great a barrier to older people as steps are to a wheelchair user" (Hiatt, 1985). Furnishings and materials that absorb sound, reduce echoes, and muffle irrelevant noise can alleviate acoustical distractions. The use of acoustical ceiling tile is usually the most economical and effective way to lower sound levels, but carpeting, draperies, and other upholstery fabrics also reduce noise levels. Decorative baffles and wall hangings reduce background noise and add aesthetic visual appeal.

In an area where incontinence may be a problem, velour-like plastics or polyester upholstery using a vapor barrier can be specified. This upholstery is installed with velcro and can be laundered in a clothes washer and line dried. This special fabric provides the texture and warmth of upholstery while still addressing the problems of maintenance.

Insulating sheetrock should be used around noisy areas, such as kitchens, maintenance and mechanical rooms. Tight window weather seals reduce exterior sound noise. On the exterior, earth berms, trees and large plant material will assist in diverting and absorbing traffic sounds in urban settings. On the other hand, sound can cue the activity room, lounge, or beauty shop.

Utilizing Taste and Smell

Taste. The sense of taste consists of four components—sweet, salty, bitter, and sour—all of which are chemically induced. It appears that changes in the gustatory system do not seriously affect the sense of taste until relatively late in life. However, medications, dentures and certain diseases have an impact on the sense of taste.

The food service department needs to consider these factors. Because so many residents have either a salt or sugar-restricted diet, the dietitian needs to find safe substitutes, such as a variety of herbs and spices, in order to provide greater food satisfaction for the older person. Gustatory stimulation can occur at tasting parties (wine, cheese, ice cream, etc.) or become a part of "redundant" cuing, when an ethnic dinner is combined with music, costumes, dances and visual effects.

Smell. The sense of smell provides protection and pleasure. It can generate associations of ideas and past experience. Aromas of fresh-mown hay and rain-soaked sod conjure up more than smells. Helen Keller utilized her keen sense of smell to identify people. Moreover, two-thirds of the response to taste is the sense of smell. The aroma of food changes mere acceptance into appreciation of flavor.

The literature on olfactory (smell) sensitivity is contradictory, but it appears to decrease with age. There is not only a reduction of pleasant smells, but a reduced sensitivity to body odors and smoke or gas fumes. In a study in England by Chalke of 892 deaths due to domestic gas poisoning, over 75 percent of the persons who died were over 60 years of age.

Opportunities to increase good smells include the smell of baking, coffee, popcorn, plants, and fresh air. Plants that are colorful and fragrant should be selected, both inside and outside the facility. In an area for confused residents, plants must be of a non-poisonous variety.

Tactile/Touch Concerns

Sensory input through the skin is subdivided into the touch and the tactile systems. Touch provides awareness and protective responses and tactile input interacts with the environment.

Tactile Input. Tactile receptors allow us to perceive multiple characteristics of an object. For example a wet rock may also be cold, hard, and smooth. When other senses are impaired, particularly vision and hearing, the older person relies more on the tactile sense. However, there are also decreases in this sense. So while discrimination is decreasing, the older person is depending more upon it. According to researchers, implications for environmental design relate to tactile discrimination.

Textures should be carefully combined in the environment so as not to overload the individual. One dominant texture in an area is more effective than many varied textures together. Coarse wall hangings made from burlap, carpet, heavy yarns, or rope will add interesting texture. Carpeting, velour, textured upholstery, and wood, not only cut down on glare, but add warmth and tactile input. Varied floor coverings likewise increase the degree of texture in an area. Outdoors, a distinctive surface treatment can lead the older person to a particular seating area.

Tactile information can also be used for other cues. Variations on the surface of handrails, such as knurling or grooves, can give cues to turns or the approaching end of a wall. Fire and exterior doorknobs are required to have some type of textural surface for safety purposes.

Older persons are more sensitive to temperature extremes. They are more likely to complain of being too cold rather than too hot. They often require lap robes and sweaters in temperatures that to the younger person seem much too warm. Outdoor environments should be protected from breezes with fences or baffles. Providing a variety of fabrics in blankets, towels, and clothing can eliminate total tactical deprivation.

Touch. Researchers have identified the need for being touched. Touch enhances the feeling of well-being, but as people age, they have fewer significant others with whom touching is acceptable behavior. "One has only to observe the responses of older people to a caress, an embrace, a hand-pat or a clasp, to appreciate how vitally necessary such experiences are for their well-being" (Montagu).

Care givers may need to learn the importance of using a caring touch with the elderly and to give and receive touch comfortably. The staff must be aware that an occasional resident may have an aversion to being touched for psychological, cultural, or social reasons. Touch levels must be comfortable for the resident.

For the seriously ill or confused, touch is a valuable communication tool. The use of touch with seriously ill patients was found to indicate that the nurse cares about them (McCorkle). "A simple warm, human gesture like a hand on his/her shoulder can do more to help an elderly regressed patient respond than many sophisticated techniques" (Burnside). Some research indicates that the dozing and inattentiveness we see in the elderly "confused" population may be fostered by a lack of touch/tactile stimulation. Touch can also be observed when residents cling to personal possessions that evoke memories (Huss).

Kinesthetic Input

Kinesthesia, the position and balance sense, has two groups of sensors. The proprioceptive sense, located in the joints and deep tissue of the limbs, indicates the position of body parts in space. Changes result in deficits in motor coordination and cause the elderly to move more slowly in shorter, higher, and wider based steps.

The second relates to balance. Changes in the vestibular system of the inner ear gives input concerning an individual's head position. Elderly persons have less ability to determine what direction the head is moving which leads to an increase in the possibility of falling (Hasselkus). Decreased strength of the postural muscles of the trunk also leads to a reduction of balance and equilibrium reactions. The younger person merely tilts forward to maintain balance. The older person is less able to determine when the body is tilting which leads to falls.

Floor Covering. Carpet has approximately the same installation price as sheet vinyl but produces more drag on the wheels which causes difficulties for some wheelchair users. Maintenance requires immediate cleaning of spills. A feeling of warmth and comfort is projected by carpet; it is quiet, traps air-born bacteria dust; and has a wide color and texture range. Residents appear to feel more secure on carpet. Gait speed and step length have been demonstrated to be significantly greater on carpet than on a vinyl surface (Willmott). Vinyl composition tile (VCT) is good for wheelchair traffic, is relatively inexpensive to install and has adequate color choices. It has high maintenance requirements, is noisy, produces glare and has an institutional appearance. Although installation costs for VCT are the least expensive, user-cost comparison shows carpet, over the lifetime of the product, to be less (Reznikoff). Another alternative is to use carpet squares in high traffic areas where they can be easily replaced at minimal expense.

Ambulation Aids. Code mandates that handrails be 32 inches on both sides of the corridor. However, observations of ambulation in nursing homes have shown that only a minority of ambulatory residents actually use the handrail for assistance while walking. The main use of the handrail is by the person in the wheelchair who pulls him/herself down the hall using the handrail to assist his/her movement. Koncelik has suggested a second handrail on the same wall, at approximately 26 inches.

The shape of the handrail should provide comfortable grasp and maximum safety. The best handrail design is cylindrical in shape and 1¼ to 1½ inches in diameter. Support should also be available in dining, activity and day rooms and tables should be sturdy because most older people will use them for support. Because of postural changes, stairs rather than ramps may be safer and easier for older people to negotiate (Hiatt, 1979). Although a ramp is a requirement for the wheelchair user, the lower gaze, combined with forward tilt due to osteoporosis and the ramp incline may alter balance for the ambulatory older person. This may tend to increase falls.

For older wheelchair users, ramps must not be too steep because of reduced upper extremity strength. The ramp for the older person should have a pitch of one foot for twenty feet of length (1:20) rather than the accessibility standard of 1:12.

Other Considerations. Tactile, kinesthetic, and vestibular stimulation have been relatively unexplored in the elderly. Even the recognition of the importance of touch at other ages is fairly recent. Research by Kramer has documented that preterm infants that were rocked mechanically on waterbeds and given auditory stimulation gained significantly more weight than nonstimulated infants. Harlow's experiments with rhesus monkeys deprived of touch and kinesthetic stimulation showed these monkeys resorted to body-rocking. This is similar to children who are raised in institutions and touched infrequently (Montagu).

Rocking behavior is commonly seen in disoriented elderly. Is this self-induced movement an attempt to increase vestibular stimulation? The need for self-determined vestibular input can be encouraged by including rocking chairs in the facility. Outdoor porches are a good investment for resident well-being, particularly if porch swings and rocking chairs are included in this area. The arm of the swing should be part of the support system of the chair and not moveable.

SUMMARY

The environment can enhance physical and mental function if supportive design interventions are provided. Many design features can increase or decrase dependence and self-esteem. For these reasons, the physical environment must be viewed as an integral part of the treatment system. It is the administrator's responsibility to increase staff sensitivity to the role of the environment and to help identify supportive and therapeutic features of the facility.

RESOURCES

American Foundation for the Blind, 15 West 16th Street, New York, New York, 10011.

American Institute of Architects. *Design for Aging: An Architect's Guide,* AIA Press, Washington D.C., 1985.

Aranyi, L. and L. Goldman. *Design of Long-Term Care Facilities,* Van Nostrand Reinhold, 1980.

Carroll, K. *The Nursing Home Environment,* Minneapolis, MN, Ebenezer Center for Aging and Human Development, 1978.

Hall, G. et al, "Sheltered Freedom, An Alzheimer's Unit in ICF", *Geriatric Nursing*, May/June, 1986, pp 132–137.

Hiatt, L. "Conveying the Substance of Images", *Contemporary Administrator*, 7(4):17–22, April 1984.

Hoglund, J. David. *Housing for the Elderly: Privacy and Independence in Environments for the Aging*, New York, Van Nostrand Reinhold Company, 1985.

Minneapolis Society for the Blind, 1936 Lyndale Avenue, South, Minneapolis, Minn. 55403 (612) 871-2222.

Wolanin, M.O. and L. R. Phillips. *Confusion; Prevention and Care*, St. Louis, Mo., C. V. Mosby, 1981.

REFERENCES

Bowersox, J., "Architectural and Interior Design", in *Long Term Care of the Aging: A Socially Responsible Approach*, ed. Lois J. Wasser, Washington, D.C., American Assoc. of Homes for the Aging, 1979.

Burnside, I.M, "Touching is Talking," *American Journal of* Nursing, *73(12):2060-2063, December 1973.*

Chalke, H. and Dewhurst, J. "Coal gas poisoning: Loss of sense of smell as a possible contributory factor with old people", *British Medical Journal* 2:1915–1917, 1957.

Cooper, B., Gowland, C., McIntosh, J. "The Use of Color in the Environment of the Elderly to Enhance Function," *Clinics in Geriatric Medicine*, 2(1):151–163, February, 1986.

Cristarella, M.C. "Visual Function of the Elderly", *American* Journal of Occupational Therapy *31(7):432-40, August,* 1977.

Gelard, F. *The Human Senses*, New York, John Wiley, Inc. 1953.

Hall, G., Kirschling, M. and Todd, S. "Sheltered Freedom, An Alzheimer's Unit in ICF," *Geriatric Nursing*, May/June, 1986.

Hasselkus, B. "Aging and the Human Nervous System," *American Journal of Occupational Therapy*, 28(1):16–21, 1974.

Hatton, J. "Aging and the glare problems", *Journal Gerontological Nursing*, 3:38–44, 1977.

Hiatt, L.G. "Architecture for the Aged: Design for Living," *Inland Architect*, 6–18, 41–42, November/December 1979. . *"Is Poor Light Dimming the Sight of Nursing Home* Patients" *Nursing Homes*, pp. 32–41, Oct. 1980.

——————— Personal Conversation, July, 1987.

——————— "The Color and Use of Color in Environments for Older People, *Nursing Homes*, 30(3):1822, 1981.

——————— "Understanding the Physical Environment," *Pride Institute Journal of Long Term Care Health Care*, 4(2):12–22, 1985.

Huss, A.J. "Touch with care or a caring touch", *American Journal of Occupational Therapy*, 31:11–18, 1977.

Koncelik, Joseph A. *Designing the Open Nursing Home*. Stroudsburg, PA, Dowden, Hutchingson & Ross, 1976.

Kramer, L. and Piermont, M. "Rocking water beds and auditory stimuli to enhance growth of preterm infants," *Journal of Pediatrics,* 88:297–299, 1976.

Lawton, M. P. *Environment and Aging,* Monterey Calif., Brooks/Cole, 1980.

Liebowitz, B., Lawton, M.P., and Waldman, A. "Evaluation: Designing for Confused Elderly People," *American Institute of Architects Journal,* 59–61, February 1979.

Montagu, A. *Touching, the Human Significance of the Skin,* New York, Harper and Row, 1974.

Parent, L. "Effect of the LOw-Stimulus Environment on Behavior," *American Journal of Occupational Therapy* 32(1):19–25, January, 1978.

Peppard, N. "A Special Nursing Home Unit," *Generations,* 9(2):62–63, Winter, 1984.

Schafer, S., "Modifying Environments," *Geriatric Nursing,* 157–159, May/June 1985.

Sicurella, V.J. "Color Contrast as an Aid for Visually Impaired Persons," *Journal of Visual Impairment and Blindness,* 72:252–257, 1977.

Snyder, L., Pyrek, J., and Smith K. "Vision and mental function of the elderly," *Gerontologist,* 16:491–495, 1976.

—————————. "Wandering," *Gerontologist,* 18:272–280, 1978.

Steffens, R. and Thralow, J., "Visual Field Limitations in the Patient with Dementia of the Alzheimer's Type," *Journal of the American Geriatrics Society* 35(3)198–204, March 1987.

Willmott, M., "The Effect of a Vinyl Floor Surface and Carpeted Floor Surface Upon Walking in Elderly." Hospital In-Patients, *Age and Aging,* 15:119–120, 1986.

CREATING THE ENVIRONMENT FOR LIVING

A dministrators of long-term care organizations have a triad of responsibilities: one, to develop a sound organization; two, to employ and
develop a team of geriatric health care specialists; and three, to enrich
day-to-day living for residents. Part V addresses the latter responsibility.

Chapter 8, Managing the Effects of Institutional Living, examined the
staff and resident outcomes of various kinds of administrative approaches
to institutions where people live over a period of time. The following
chapters suggest more specific ways of humanizing the environment,
ways of increasing affectional bonds.

Chapter 19, Families: The Second Client, discusses ways of helping
families to maintain their ties throughout the institutional stay. Chapter 20, Children in the Environment, discusses ways of increasing intergenerational relationships, and Chapter 21, Companion Animals in the
Environment, explores the bonds between people and pets as a bridge to
improved interpersonal relationships. Finally, Chapter 22, Care of the
Dying Among Friends, suggests ways of helping both staff and residents
to deal with the inevitable event of death.

Chapter 19

FAMILIES: THE SECOND CLIENT

CAROL WOEHRER AND RUTH STRYKER

INTRODUCTION

The long-term care administrator's role is highly unusual in that s/he is not only responsible for coordinating and leading effective and efficient provision of typical health services but also for facilitating the maintenance, development, and enrichment of expressive and emotional relationships. To minimize the negative effects of institutionalization discussed in Chapter 8, the long-term care administrator must give special attention to the development of systems, policies, and programs that foster caring informal relationships between residents, families, and employees. The kind of systems, policies, and programs to promote and maintain familial ties is the subject of this chapter.

CONTEMPORARY INTERGENERATIONAL RELATIONS

It is sometimes assumed that older people go to long-term care facilities because families nowadays are less close and less willing to care for older parents in the home as in days past. Although there are differences among ethnic groups, socioeconomic groups, rural and urban settings, and individual relationships, ties of commitment and obligation remain strong between generations in the American family, and the family remains a strongly supportive institution for the older person (Neugarten, 1979). A rosy glorification of the past only serves to infuse the contemporary family with guilt and disappointment (Treas, 1979).

Historical evidence indicates that the three-generation household was never very popular and existed mainly for financial reasons. Recent attitude studies indicate that both younger and older people also favor independent living arrangements. Though most older people prefer to live independently, they do turn to their children when in need of assistance (Brody, 1977; Neugarten, 1975; Riley and Foner, 1968; Troll, 1971). Most older people live near at least one of their children, see one of their children weekly, and receive household help in time of illness from them (Kerchoff, 1965; Rosenberg, 1970; Rosow, 1967; Sussman, 1965; Hill, 1970). By the same token, adult children turn to their parents in time of need.

While independence governed intergenerational living arrangements both in the past and the present, it is more common for single elderly people to live with kin. Approximately one-third of single people over the age of sixty-five currently live with kin (Mindel, 1979), a drop since 1950. The decline is due to the greater affluence of today's elderly and to the fact that many contemporary older people had smaller families during the depression. This trend is likely to continue because 1) more aged will have elderly children, 2) more middle-aged women are working, 3) there are a greater number of four and five generation families than ever before, and 4) current birth rates are low.

Children strive to delay their parents' institutionalization, often at considerable cost to themselves (Shanas, 1979; Wershow, 1976) and living with a relative often precedes an older person's entry into a long-term care facility. Indeed, about 80 percent of all home care is provided by families. Arranging for an elderly relative to live in a facility is usually the last rather than the first resort of families (Brody, 1977). The relocation of a parent or parent-in-law often does not occur suddenly but follows a lengthy period of steady mental and physical deterioration which taxes the middle-aged child's ability to cope with the situation (Robinson and Thurnher, 1979: Brody, 1985).

The importance of family care is dramatized by the fact that persons over sixty-five living in a long-term care facility are three times as likely never to have been married and twice as likely to be widowed as older persons in the community (Shanas, 1979b). About 10 percent of long-term care residents are married in comparison to 54 percent of the elderly in the community.

When a spouse or daughter is available as caregiver, the caregiving role can involve excessive stress without the support of additional family members or friends. It is very important that the caregiver be relieved from time to time and have opportunities for frequent social interaction with sympathetic friends and relatives.

In a study of older persons with chronic brain syndrome, contrary to expectations, the extent of cognitive impairment, the frequency of memory and behavior problems, the level of functional impairment, and the duration of the illness were not related to feelings of burden by the primary caregiver. Only the frequency of family visits was related to the level of burden. Respondents receiving more visits from children, grandchildren, and siblings reported less burden (Zarit et al., 1980). Gordon's study showed that the greater the size of the household, the greater the willingness to care for an aging relative. It seems more and more evident that caregivers need support themselves (1987).

The situation of the potential caregiver influences the ability to provide care to aging parents in the community. It is the old-old, those eighty and over, who are most likely to be in need of care. Their increasing dependency needs often occur at a time when the potential caregivers are experiencing major life transitions. Adult children in middle age and early old age may be facing retirement, loss of income, lower energy levels, sensory declines, chronic ailments, and the deaths of friends, spouses, and siblings. In addition, the needs of children and grandchildren may compete for their time, energy, and financial resources.

Participation in the labor force makes it even more difficult for women to carry out their traditional caregiving role. Over half of wives forty-five to fifty-four are in the labor force. A recent study comparing the percentage of community care of mentally impaired older persons in several communities shows that community care is inversely related to the percent of women in the work force (Nardone, 1980).

In addition, family values also influence decisions regarding health care. In some families, for example, interdependence between family members is highly valued and close family relationships take precedence over activities and relationships outside the family. In other families, independence between generations is emphasized, and individuals value a high level of community participation. In our pluralistic society, with people of many different backgrounds, families vary a great deal, and these variations tend to follow ethnic cultural patterns.

It should also be noted that family relationships are never benign. Sibling rivalries, resentment from perceived or real childhood neglect or abuses, and varying levels of maturity during twenty years of living together culminate in very complex family dynamics and behaviors. Adult children may assist their parents grudgingly or with great warmth and affection. Some may not participate in care at all and a few may be abusers themselves. The Vulnerable Adults Protection Acts (enacted in most states) act to protect adults from abuse both in institutions and at home. Each resident of a nursing home and the resident's family will be unique. Lifetime patterns will not alter and staff must learn that there is no "typical" family.

THE FAMILY AS CLIENT

The admission of an individual to a long-term care facility is a time of crisis for both the resident and the family. The aged person must cope with loss of independence and feelings of rejection. The children experience feelings of failure, guilt, and anguish as they observe declines in the physical and mental health of aging parents. Family members will react to anxiety and conflict in a number of ways. Some overzealously attempt to take care of everything themselves to the point of nervous exhaustion. Others avoid the situation and stay away from parents. Some vascillate between approach and avoidance, carrying on until they cannot tolerate further pressure, switching subsequently to avoidance. The most successful in dealing with increasing parental dependence are those who realistically do what they can and seek support and help from other kin and community services (Steinman, 1979).

Organizations must balance their approach to family programming from a variety of perspectives; 1) for the good of the resident with family services contributing to higher morale, 2) helping staff to achieve greater job meaning through their work with families and 3) meeting the needs of families, regarding them as clients of the facility.

When staff and families maintain open communications, there are multiple opportunities to develop mutual understanding as to what staff are attempting to accomplish and how they are proceeding. When families express appreciation and support for staff, it is very rewarding. When a resident exhibits behavior that is difficult to manage, a family conference can be called to "explore causes as well as ways families have best dealt with such behaviors." Staff must then express their gratitude for such assistance. If there is dissention within a family or there is disagreement between family and staff, primary care givers must attempt to resolve care problems with families in order to serve the best interests of residents, families and staff.

The three perspectives regarding families, as provider of service to residents, as support to staff, and as a second client all have merit. This chapter, however, encourages long-term care administrators to focus on the family as client because doing so not only best meets the needs of families, but also optimizes family support of both residents and staff.

In a comparison of three long-term care facilities, Rhonda Montgomery found that homes that viewed the family as a client had the highest family participation in terms of number of visits to residents, attendance at events, and performance of helping tasks, whereas the facility which viewed the family as a provider of services to residents had the least participation. The home with no family programming and policies ranked between. In the home which encouraged a client role, residents and families consulted more frequently and considered the family as a whole in decision making.

When a facility fosters a service role for the family, the resident's good is viewed as receiving priority. This places the staff and resident against the family and results in considerable family withdrawal. Interestingly, fostering a service role for the family fosters dependence in the resident, one who needs to be served. A client role for the family, on the other hand, encourages the acceptance of responsibility by the residents. Since both residents and families are viewed as having needs, decisions reflect the wider family good. Residents perceive themselves as having continuing influence on family members.

By fostering families as clients, family members develop the self-acceptance, knowledge, and skills they need to interact in a way which is more rewarding to both the resident and themselves. Family philosophy, programming, and policies cover four areas: (1) helping family members to accept feelings surrounding the entrance of a relative to the facility; (2) clarification of continuing family responsibilities of the resident in the facility; (3) information regarding the facility's services, resources, and policies; (4) development of primary relationships for those residents who have few or no close family members or friends.

CREATING A FACILITY-WIDE APPROACH

Making family members feel at home in the facility and helping them define their role in relationship to the resident requires a facility-wide approach. This does not happen unless the administrator assumes leadership by setting expectations. The best social worker cannot compensate for staff members who are indifferent to families or regard them as interfering with the routines of the facility. Her warm welcome will seem hollow if families confront restricted visiting hours or institutional red tape. First, facility policies and procedures need to be assessed for impact on family and friends' abilities to relate to residents. Some will not be needed at all.

Whether they do so to the benefit or detriment of residents and families depends on their knowledge, sensitivity, and skill. Staff members, even with the best of intentions, may obstruct family relationships. It is not unusual for relatives and friends to be made to feel unwanted by nurses or aides who look away and ignore their presence, for family members to be made to feel guilty by staff members who regard themselves as residents' advocates, and for family members to feel they are inadequate by staff members who complain about the inconvenience they cause. The influence of staff members on families should not be left to chance. With proper training all staff members can become advocates of both residents and families and can contribute to enriching residents' social relationships.

As Dubrof points out, all staff members should receive training related to family relationships. Switchboard operators and receptionists located near the facility entrance often witness encounters that other staff do not. The mail sorter and distributor may notice disruptions in patterns of communication between an older person and family members. Housekeepers often develop informal relationships with residents and have frequent interaction with their friends and relatives. Activities staff hopefully include family members in programs and recruit them as volunteers. And nurses and nursing assistants, particularly those on duty during evening shifts and weekends, encounter families most regularly. While the amount and depth of training will vary with the job, some training is needed by all employees.

The administrator can evaluate the adequacy of staff training in relating to families as a second client by reviewing the organization's orientation and inservice programs. The orientation and inservice education of staff members should include content on (1) relationships of residents without families, (2) the needs and feelings of family members, (3) the impact of staff attitudes and behavior on family relationships, (4) the effects of memory loss on relationships, (5) communication with residents and their friends and relatives, and (6) the resource persons for concerns regarding social relationships or the well-being of the resident.

In general, long-term care residents have fewer close family members than older people in the community. However, in some small towns, almost all residents have relatives and friends close by while in the inner cities, 80 percent or more of the residents may have no relatives living in the vicinity. Programming to meet the psychosocial needs of residents should be developed within the context of the wider social worlds of a facility's residents.

Staff members also need to be educated regarding the stress and feelings of unhappiness, loneliness, guilt, anxiety, and alienation that families and friends experience when the health of someone they care for declines and entry to a long-term care facility becomes necessary. They need to understand what they can do to alleviate these feelings. Listening skills, a nonjudgmental approach to families, a warm welcome, and staff encouragement of families and friends are essential. The administrator should require department heads to include responsibilities for meeting the psychosocial needs of residents and families in job descriptions, and provide instruction to supervisors and department heads on how to evaluate employees on this aspect of their positions. In staff training sessions, it is very helpful to have family members and residents explain what they found stressful in long-term care placement and living in the facility and what things staff did that helped them deal with stress and anxiety to make them feel at ease.

Staff training sessions cannot deal with all possible circumstances and situations that employees will face. Therefore, an important component is to provide resources when concerns arise. Many residents experience memory loss and thus complain that sons or daughters have not visited for a long time even when they visited the same day. On hearing such a complaint, it is natural for employees to feel concerned, and it should be checked out both to enable the facility to meet residents and families' needs and to help the employee understand the situation. Conversely, a confused resident may report not having a bath or meal to a family member who then raises the issue with staff. Staff members must then check to see whether there was an omission of care. This may involve checking records or talking with a receptionist, social worker, or a nursing employee on an overlapping shift.

To assure that families and friends are a part of facility life, administrators must encourage efforts by key staff members: the social worker, the activities director, and the director of nursing.

The director of nursing must insure that family responsibilities are included in job descriptions, supervision, policies and employee evaluations. The activity director's responsibilities should include the development of activities in which family members, friends, and children can participate and the coordination of special events for families and friends. The administrator should require the activities department to offer programs appropriate for family participation evenings and weekends when family members visit most frequently.

A commitment to serving family needs is likely to wither through indifference or possible subversion without strong administrative support and continuous monitoring. The administrator, director of nursing, activities director, and social worker serve as staff models when they are observed with family members. They should not only be available to families but actively seek family contact by being available for one evening per week or two weekend afternoons per month, depending on families' needs.

Discovering and Developing the Residents' Social Network

Research on social aspects of aging indicates that it is not the number of social activities or friends an older person has that has the greatest influence on morale. Rather, it is the depth and meaning of the relationship that makes a significant difference. A person who has a confidant is less likely to become depressed even if overall social interaction decreases than one who has no confidant, but high social interaction (Lowenthal and Haven, 1968). What this suggests is that facilities can have the greatest impact on the emotional well-being of residents by facilitating the maintenance and development of relationships with confidants.

The social worker must assess the resident's social network so that significant people continue to be a part of the resident's life in the facility. Families can help as part of a family orientation program. The task is to discover the people with whom the older person interacted, the frequency and significance of the interaction, and the mode of interaction. Because of lack of transportation and difficulty in walking long distances, many older people are not able to get together frequently with friends and relatives. Many residents, maintain contact with friends and relatives by a phone in the room. Families should be encouraged to make this a high priority if the resident is able to use a phone.

A high percentage of long-term care residents do not have spouses or children. However, many do have brothers, sisters, cousins, nieces, and nephews with whom they have been in frequent contact. For these residents, neighbors can sometimes be helpful in locating close friends and relatives. When a support network is not apparent, staff members should be alerted to listen to the resident talk about friends and relatives and inform the social worker if they hear of people that might be contacted.

It is not unusual, of course, for residents in long-term care facilities to have no social network or a very weak one. Staff members may become the surrogate family for these residents. Because a confidant is especially important for people's morale, the resident might be introduced to another with a similar language, profession, area of the country, disability, interests, or outlook on life. Or it might be suggested that a resident help another in some way: by pushing a wheelchair, demonstrating a crochet stitch, or writing a letter. Staff members and volunteers, can be assigned on a one-to-one basis to spend time with residents who do not have their own natural social network. A foster grandparent program could also help these residents.

Creating a social network is most difficult for those residents who have memory loss. Since recent memory is generally lost first, long-term relationships are easier to maintain than new ones are to create. With a warm accepting atmosphere and a sympathetic sense of humor, it is possible to help residents with chronic brain syndrome relate to others through memory loss support groups and validation therapy. The development of relationships does depend on memory, however. For residents with severe memory loss, perhaps the best that staff can do is to provide frequent hugs and reassurance.

Strengthening the Organization's Commitment to Families

Recent studies indicate that family relationships can not only be maintained, but enriched in the long-term care setting. A study in California reflected a continuation or improvement in family relationships following placement in a well-regarded long-term care facility. Thirty percent of families experienced renewed closeness or strengthening of family ties, 15 percent a discovery of new love and affection, 25 percent continuation of closeness, 20 percent continuation of separateness, and 10 percent frequent interaction without quality. Family members cited the alleviation of preadmission strains, the physical and/or mental improvement displayed by the parent following institutionalization, and the parent's involvement with other residents as reasons for the strengthening of family relationships (Smith and Bengtson, 1979).

Most families do not "put grandma away." They expect to continue to have a part in her life. Through its policies and programs, however, the long-term care facility can recruit family members and enrich family relationships, or it can discourage family members.

One way the administrator can strengthen commitment to family involvement is through the development of a family council. The family council is a group of friends and relatives of nursing home residents. The purpose of the family council is to promote understanding of the organization, family participation in planning and decision making, and family contribution to quality of life in the long-term care facility. The goals and functions of the family council may include (1) policy and planning input to administrative decision making through evaluation of current programs and policies and suggestions for changes, (2) aid to families of current and prospective residents through information and support, (3) direction and recommendations for the content of family programming within the facility, (4) contribution of volunteer expertise and skills, and (5) advocacy for nursing home residents through pursuit of change in the facility or in legislative or regulatory areas (Boyle and Kauffman, 1981).

Usually only a small number of family members, perhaps one for every ten residents, participates in a family council since it involves a greater commitment of time. These dedicated family members, however, can become a very effective and invaluable liaison between families, residents, and administration. The administrator can contribute to their effectiveness by allocating staff time through social services for organizing and coordinating the council; by providing opportunities for family council members to gain knowledge and understanding of the home's operation through meetings with department heads and representatives of regulatory and funding agencies; by responding to council questions, suggestions, and concerns; and by attending family council meetings which involve administrative issues and facility-wide policies.

SUMMARY

Family involvement in the long-term care organization requires active initiation of systems, programs and policies, continuous monitoring, and evaluation by the administrator. The goals of family involvement are to maintain and enhance family relationships, to support families, and to facilitate family influence on the organization's policies and programs. Because families relate to many different employees, a facility-wide approach is required. Therefore, the administrator should select employees with sensitivity to families from the social services, nursing, activities, and perhaps other departments to serve as a committee for the development and implementation of a facility-wide approach.

Since family members and friends are a natural and invaluable resource for the psychological well-being and happiness of residents, time spent on facilitating family involvement can bring multiple benefits with minimal costs. Nevertheless, the development and implementation of family communication systems and programs does take time. It is essential that the administrator place a high priority on these responsibilities by allocating sufficient time for staff to carry them out.

Staff responsibilities can be designated through job descriptions. Family involvement, staff responsibilities, and standards for interaction with families need to be monitored. Monitoring does not require extensive resources, but it does require diligence. The administrator should review the communication system for family involvement as well as the system for supervision of staff relations with residents and families.

Finally, it is important for the administrator to evaluate the impact of communication systems, policies, and programs on families and residents' relationships to their families. Records should be kept on questions and problems in order to look for patterns in questions, problems, or concerns. These patterns can indicate a need for changes in policies or programs, for employee education, or for additional information in resident or family handbooks. The family council can also be an excellent resource for giving feedback on how families are relating to the organization and what impact the facility is having on them.

It is essential for the administrator to remember that the goal of the organization's family policies and programs is the enhancement of the informal relationships between residents and families. This goal is less tangible than the more instrumental goals of keeping the home clean, giving rehabilitative therapy to maximize resident's independence, and providing nutritious meals. As a less tangible goal, it is harder to measure and easier to lose sight of. Nonetheless, it is vital for the well-being and happiness of both clients.

REFERENCES

Boyle, Gayle M. and Kauffman, Barbara K. *Family Councils in Nursing Homes.* Minneapolis, Ebenezer Center for Aging and Human Development, 1981.

Brody, Elaine M. *Long Term Care of Older People: A Practical Guide.* New York, Human Sciences Press, 1977.

Brody, Elaine M. "Parent Care as a normative Family Stress." *The Gerontologist,* 25:1:19–29, 1985.

Dubrof, Rose, and Eugene Litwak. *Maintenance of Family Ties of Long Term Care Patients.* U.S. Department of Health, Education and Welfare, DHEW Publication No. (ADM) 77-400, 1977.

Gordon, George Kenneth. *Family Size and Intent to Care for Elderly Relatives,* unpublished study, University of Minnesota, 1987.

Hill, Reuben. *Development in Three Generations.* Cambridge, MA, Schenkman Publishing Company, 1970.

Kerchoff, A.C. "Nuclear and Extended Family Relationships" in Ethel Shanas and Gordon Streib (Eds), *Social Structure and Family: Generational Relations,* Englewood Cliffs, NJ, Prentice-Hall, 1965.

Lowenthal, M. F. and C. Haven. "Interaction and Adaptation: Intimacy as a Critical Variable" in Bernice Neugarten (Ed) *Middle Age and Aging,* Chicago, University of Chicago Press, 1968.

Mindel, Charles H. Multigenerational Family Households: Recent Trends and Implications for the Future. *Gerontologist, 19,* 5, October, 1979, pp. 456–463.

Montgomery, Rhonda Jean Voigt. *Relationships of Residents of Long Term Health Care Institutions to Their Families and Staff.* Dissertation, University of Minnesota, 1980.

Nardone, Maryann. Characteristics Predicting Community Care for Mentally Impaired Older Persons. *Gerontologist, 20,* 6, 1980, pp. 661–668.

Neugarten, Bernice L. The Middle Generations. In Pauline K. Ragan (Ed.), *Aging Parents.* Los Angeles, University of Southern California Press, 1979.

Neugarten, Bernice L. (Ed.). Aging in the Year 2000: A Look at the Future. *Gerontologist, 15,* 1975, pp. 1–40.

Riley, M. W., and Foner, A. *Aging and Society, Volume 1: An Inventory of Research Findings.* New York, Russell Sage Foundation, 1968.

Robinson, Betsy, and Thurnher, Majda. Taking Care of Aged Parents: A Family Cycle Transition, *Gerontologist, 19,* 6, 1979, pp. 586–593.

Rosenberg, G. S. *The Worker Grows Old.* San Francisco, Jossey-Bass, 1970.

Rosow, Irving. *Social Integration of the Aged.* New York, Free Press, 1967.

Shanas, Ethel. The Family as a Social Support System in Old Age, *Gerontologist, 19,* 2, 1979a, pp. 169–174.

Shanas, Ethel. Social Myth as Hypothesis: The Case of the Family Relations of Old People, *Gerontologist, 19,* 1, 1979b, pp. 3–9.

Smith, Kristen Felde and Bengtson, Vern L. Positive Consequences of Institutionalization: Solidarity Between Elderly Parents and Their Middle-Aged Children, *Gerontologist, 19,* 5, 1979, pp. 438–447.

Soldo, Beth J. and Jaana Myllyluoma. "Caregivers Who Live with Dependen Elderly," *The Gerontologist,* 23:6:605–611, 1983.

Steinman, Lynne A. "Reactivated Conflicts with Aging Parents" in Pauline K Ragan (Ed) *Aging Parents,* Los Angeles, CA, University of Southern California Press, 1979.

Sussman, Marvin B. "Relationships of Adult Children with Their Parents in the U.S." in Ethel Shanas and Gordon Streib (eds) *Social Structure and the Family: Generational Relations,* Englewood Cliffs, NJ, Prentice-Hall, 1965.

Tobin, Sheldon and Regina Kulys. "Older People and Their Responsible Others," *Social Work,* pp. 138–145, March 1983.

Treas, Judith. "Intergenerational Families and Social Change" in Pauline K. Ragan (Ed) *Aging Parents,* Los Angeles, University of Southern California Press, 1979.

Troll, Lillian E. "The Family of Later Life:A Decade Review," *Journal of Marriage and the Family,* 33:263–290, 1971.

Wershow, H. J. "The Four Percent Fallacy:Some Further Evidence and Political Implications," *The Gerontologist,* 16:1:52–55, 1976.

York, Jonathan L. and Robert J. Calsyn. "Family Involvement in Nursing Homes," *The Gerontologist,* 17:6:500–505, 1977.

Zarit, Steven H., Karen E. Reever and Julie Bach-Peterson, "Relatives of the Imaered Elderly: Correlates of Feelings of Burden," *The Gerontologist,* 20:6:649–655, 1980.

RECOMMENDED READINGS

Blodgett, Harriet E., Evelyn Deno, and Virginia Hathaway. *For the Caregivers: Caring for Patients with Brain Loss,* Minneapolis, University of Minnesota Press, 1985.

Cohen, Donna and Carl Eisdorfer. *The Loss of Self,* New York, Nal Penguin Inc., 1986.

Mace, N.L. and P.V. Rabins. *The 36-Hour Day:A Family Guide for Persons with Alzheimer's Disease,* Baltimore, MD, Johns Hopkins University Press, 1981.

Troll, Lillian. *Family Issues in Current Gerontology,* New York, Springer Publishers, 1986.

Chapter 20

CHILDREN IN THE ENVIRONMENT

John Thompson and Ruth Stryker

INTRODUCTION

R esidential and recreational patterns of many contemporary American families tend to isolate the young from the old. Young people are missing the nurture, support, and sense of roots that grandparents provide. Older persons are missing the valued joy from youthful perspectives and the self esteem that comes from the role of generativity.

If this is a loss for persons living in the community, it is even more exaggerated for persons living in nursing homes where many previous psychosocial supports are reduced. Research of long-term care organizations has helped to identify characteristics that improve quality of life. As a result, long-term care facilities have learned how to better integrate the residential, psychosocial, and medical parameters of programming.

Even though new knowledge is available, stereotyped and traditional notions about the limitations of the elderly in nursing homes abound. As a result, the more vulnerable residents are deprived of many opportunities for normalcy. Long-term care facilities tend to create an overprotective atmosphere. Public expectations have been molded by standards of care which emphasize "doing for" residents. Comfort has been a goal while stimulation and growth were saved for the more energetic segment of our population. All of this results in the removal of many facets of normal living from institutional living.

WHY INTERGENERATIONAL RELATIONS?

It is the administrator's responsibility to initiate programs that encourage interpersonal relationships, especially with persons from the community. One way to do this is through intergenerational programs which can be rewarding to both nursing home residents and children. It is a way to reintroduce a chance for growth, an opportunity for emotional ties and natural exposure to a part of the real world where risk is a companion of enrichment.

More specifically, what are some of the purposes and goals of a program for intergenerational interaction? There are many. First, children are an everyday part of life in a normal community. Long-term care facilities create an artificial environment if they remove factors in the "real world" in order to protect residents, but from just what is not clear. Reminders of normalcy? Misplaced ideas that children are a bother? Dislike of noise? By not only permitting but encouraging intergenerational interactions, at least one area of community life is brought back into the residents' environment.

Second, the positive results of introduction of interaction between the old and the young comes from the innocent perceptions of the very young about the old. Children, especially those of preschool age, have not yet learned to value a person on the basis of physical or mental perfection. That trait has been saved for those of us who are too old to retain the wonder of life and yet too young to understand it. Young children do not allow wrinkles and infirmities to interfere with their relationships to others.

The third reason focuses on the spontaneous fun and humor that young children bring to any environment. Children, especially the very young with their curiosity and openness, can change the normally quiet (and often dull) institution into a vibrant and gleeful community.

Fourth, because so many affectional ties of the elderly have been broken by death or separation, children provide new ties which can fill a much-needed void. Finally, a well thought-out program can and should have a positive influence on attitudes toward the aged in future generations.

TYPES OF INTERGENERATIONAL PROGRAMS

Virtually every long-term care facility has, as a part of daily life, some interaction with children. Grandchildren and great-grandchildren are at least occasional visitors to their elderly family members. Not infrequently older grandchildren are employees of the facility where a grandparent lives.

Beyond this, programs vary greatly. Children from a local school may have a "special" friend whom they visit weekly during the school year.

A nursing home may be connected to a facility for mentally retarded children who are nurtured and helped on a one-to-one basis by frail elderly. A children's day care center may be attached to or associated with a nursing home so that relationships develop over time. Special programs for grandchildren of residents can make such visits "more fun." Grandparents may "baby sit" grandchildren for one or two hours a week. More able residents of some nursing homes even go to class with school-aged children, sitting in on their study sessions and assisting teachers in areas of their special knowledge and talent.

Many facilities are participating in foster grandparent programs. This type of approach allows school-age youngsters to develop a relationship with a resident and hopefully, a friendship. In order for a foster grandparent program to be effective, that is, to offer an opportunity for a meaningful relationship to develop, a great deal of planning and evaluation must be done. As structure increases, spontaneity decreases. Without spontaneity the mutual needs of two people can only be met by guesswork and within the confines of a pre-established program. The latter of course assumes that most people respond in a similar manner to a given set of circumstances.

The Benedictine Health Care Center in Duluth, Minnesota, built a Children's Day Care Center adjacent to the nursing home. Each child has a special friend in the nursing home. At a certain time, several days a week, the child visits the special friend. Both generations look forward to these visits. This program, while having structure, promotes spontaneous activities between friends and fosters affectional bonds that are mutually beneficial and enjoyed by both the child and the resident.

Generations Together, a part of the University of Pittsburgh Center for Social and Urban Research, has developed and studied several innovative programs. They have two major goals: 1) to improve psychosocial and physical conditions of nursing home residents and/or elderly persons in the community, and 2) to increase students' learning about aging and older persons (Newman and Lyons).

In one of their programs, a community college instructor of a psychology of aging course screened and selected ten students for weekly nursing home visits. Each student was matched with two residents who elected to participate in the program. At the end of the semester, residents reported the following positive effects:

100%— enjoyed the visits
42%— reported greater friendliness toward roommates
59%— said they left their rooms more often
41%— reported more positive feelings toward young people
88%— would recommend the program to other residents

At the end of the program, the positive results from the student interviews were:

80%— said they were more accepting of aging, their own aging, and nursing homes
70%— reported being friendlier with older persons, including their own grandparents

Several expressed an interest in a geriatric or gerontological career.

Generations Together also developed a community program called Older Friends to Children with Special Needs (Lyons and Newman). Older persons in the community volunteered time in special education classes serving retarded children. They spent time encouraging and praising children as they tried to learn. Teachers noted that the youngsters were better motivated to learn because of the special personal relationships and found that the children improved both social and physical skills. The volunteers reported improved self-esteem from contributing to others and a more openness to new ideas and experiences.

It is evident that children are a part of the lives of many elderly in the community and in some nursing homes. There have been, however, varying degrees of success depending on many variables, such as age, timeliness, frequency and access. Another variable is the degree of structure. As structure increases, spontaneity decreases. In addition, relationships develop; they cannot be forced. If either force or too much structure occurs, the program will have limited effectiveness and may even be harmful.

AN UNSTRUCTURED PROGRAM

Most long-term care organizations welcome groups of school children. During the nine-month school year, entire grades often come to visit, to entertain and hopefully to break the routine of institutional living. But does it? Watching an amateur performance of a grandchild is quite different from watching young strangers. Do these well-meaning events with children, kept at a social distance, serve to frustrate and remind the resident of his or her minimal contacts with others in the community?

And what effect does it have on the children in terms of their feelings about the aged and aging? Does seeing a room full of white haired strangers in wheelchairs create a fear of the aged and aging? Is it not better to know someone well than to have no knowledge of anyone?

These were the questions on the administrator's mind one cool fall afternoon when a school bus unloaded forty children at the entrance to the Retirement Center of Wright County, a skilled nursing facility in Buffalo, Minnesota. This was supposed to be a special day because the second grade of the elementary school was visiting.

The residents were waiting for their arrival in a large dayroom. Soon the echoes of children's chatter and giggles filled the normally quieter hallways. Then, a few songs later, the teacher ushered the children back into the bus and all was quiet again. There was an empty feeling as the residents slowly returned to their routines: television, games and naps. For a moment the atmosphere was transformed but as the children left they took with them a spark that made life more natural and exciting. The facility had reacquainted the residents with sights and sounds of children, but at the same time it seemed more like a parade. The children were only to be admired and enjoyed from a distance as if in a glass case. There was no warmth, no sharing, no relationships developed. An occasional knarled hand reached out, but the allotted time was over—for another month.

It occurred to the administrator that if children were there more—daily—and if they were the same children, this void could be filled. Coincidentally at this same time, a need for a day care center for children was becoming increasingly obvious in the community. Why not have a day care center in the nursing home?

After many months of planning with the community, state agencies, staff, residents and families, the Generations Day Care Center opened its doors in September 1979 with twenty-three children ages six weeks to twelve years old. The philosophy and premise of this Center was based on the assumption that both residents and children would mutually benefit from the opportunity to interact with each other. Since then, the original assumption of benefit has been demonstrated over and over again.

There were a great many considerations in designing and implementing a day care center for children in a long-term care facility. Costs, space, staffing, licensing according to state rules, programming and supplies and furnishings were all addressed. Through efforts by a group of dedicated volunteers, the necessary funds were raised for initial purchases and start-up costs. A director for the center was hired and applications for enrollment were taken.

Today it is the spontaneous interaction that is the magical stuff of the children's day care program. The wheelchair rides, hugs, stories and occasional tears coupled with the obvious smiles and laughs provide an atmosphere of enrichment and growth for both age groups. The halls hold evidence of real life.... a cane propped on the handlebars of a tricycle, mysterious muddy footprints appearing near the kitchen, an occasional "lost" child—usually found later on the lap of a gray-haired story-telling "kidnapper."

The community has benefitted from having a day care center and most certainly, the facility's image in the community has changed. No longer is it just a "place for old sick people." Young parents are realizing that neither the facility nor its residents are depressing as they once thought. They also find that the children are eager to return to the surroundings because of the genuine appreciation the residents have for them.

The employees benefit also. The parents of children who are employed in the nursing home have found the arrangement secure and loving. They have total access to their children and actually have a part in their lives while carrying out their employment duties. As a bonus, they have developed new dimensions to relationships with residents because of their children. Residents and employees have more to share with one another. By the same token, the child and parent have something else to share.

A number of the same children have been at the Center for some years. As a result, residents have participated daily in their growth, from baby bottles to baseball. The children have had an "extra" person who loves them and one to love. When a child loses a friend, it is dealt with openly and his or her grief is supported by others who are also saddened. As one parent said, "An introduction to death and grief is a reality with which we all must learn to deal. It is better that their first experience is with a loving friend and the support of many persons."

Today the children are a normal part of everyday life at the nursing home, but compared to several years ago, it is neither routine or structured. As one resident put it, "I can't imagine living in a place where there were no children. . . . you just can't talk to old people every minute of every day." The magic of curious children does make a difference.

REFERENCES

Bengston, V. L. and J. F. Robertson, Ed. *Grandparenthood,* Beverly Hills, CA. Sage, 1985.

Cherlin, Andrew and Frank Furstenberg. "Grandparents & Family Crisis," *Generations* X:4:26–29, Summer 1986.

Hook, W. F. et al. "Frequency of Visitation in Nursing Homes: Patterns of Contact Across the Boundaries of Total Institutions," *The Gerontologist,* 22:4:424–429, August 1982.

Kidwell, Jane I. and Booth, Alan. "Social Distance and Intergenerational Relations," *Gerontologist,* 17:5:412–420, October 1977.

Kivnick, Helen Q. "Grandparenthood: An Overview of Meaning and Mental Health," *Gerontologist, 22:*59–66, February 1982.

Lyons, Charles and Sally Newman. "Generations Together," *Generations,* X:4:29–31, Summer 1986.

Newman, Sally et al. "The Development of an Intergenerational Service-Learning Program at a Nursing Home," *The Gerontologist,* 25:2:130–133, April, 1985.

Chapter 21

COMPANION ANIMALS IN THE ENVIRONMENT

GEARY W. OLSEN, JOSEPH S. QUIGLEY AND RUTH STRYKER

In 1897 Charles Darwin stated that the American people were a "nation of pet keepers." His observation still holds true. Currently, fifty percent of American households have at least one pet, and there are approximately 60 million dogs and cats with an additional eight million horses in this country.

The word "pet" usually connotes either a dog or a cat but it may also include birds, horses, turtles, rabbits, guinea pigs, hamsters, gerbils, farm animals (used for 4-H exhibits such as goats, calves and sheep) as well as many other types of animals. People have varying degrees of emotional attachment to their animals. To express the important relationship between many humans and animals, the authors prefer to use the term "companion animal."

Companion animals are becoming recognized as a potential source of assistance in special situations. For some blind people the seeing eye dog has been an integral part of their lives as is the hearing dog for many deaf persons. More recently, there is a greater awareness of the multitude of ways in which companion animals can assist other handicapped people. The use of horses and dogs for paraplegics; monkeys for quadriplegics; and various types of companion animals for the mentally ill, emotionally disturbed and the incarcerated of our society are examples. The "Bird Man of Alcatraz" is a true example of birds having a direct positive effect on certain inmates of a prison.

Another area of recent interest is the utilization of companion animals with both the community and institutionalized elderly. However, acceptance of the value of companion animals has not always been (nor is it still) completely accepted by many people. For many years companion animals were not allowed in public housing and institutions for the elderly. The reasons given included disease transmission, behavior problems of animals, hygiene factors, the possibility of being bitten or scratched and fear that they might fall over the animals. Such fears increased the likelihood of widows or widowers, who, upon placement in a health care institution, are psychologically traumatized by giving up a beloved dog or cat, often the only remaining emotional bond after the death of loved ones.

In 1792 the York Retreat, an institution for the mentally ill in England, produced the first written documentation of using animals to improve patients' self-control through responsibility for the animals that were dependent upon them. (1) Unfortunately, over 150 years elapsed before companion animals were again used as a potential therapeutic agent for people.

In the 1960's Boris Levinson, a New York psychologist, wrote many articles including his text **Pets and Human Development** which described the role of companion animals in various stages of human development. (2) He identified the fact that a companion animal may serve as a bridge between the reluctant patient and his therapist. Levinson used his own dog as the initiator of contact between him and many of his child patients. He termed his dog a "co-therapist."

Levinson also investigated the use of companion animals with institutionalized elderly. He stated that for many elderly in nursing home environments there was no longer an incentive for further growth in their lives and that they concentrated on the past because the present was dull and the future foreboding. Levinson believed that the elderly residents' greatest source of frustration was within themselves and that they displayed fragile defense structures which could be easily traumatized. Levinson stated that a companion animal was a warranted component in many of their lives because a companion animal does not care if its master is elderly or physically handicapped. The animal may also bridge the period of readjustment to a new environment for the elderly as the animal symbolizes tranquility and stability in such a stage of turmoil.

During this same period, Corson and Corson investigated the utilization of dogs at the Ohio State Psychiatric Hospital and a nursing home in Millesburg, Ohio. (3) (4) In both instances they concluded that residents showed improvement with this form of therapy, which they labeled pet-facilitated therapy. According to the Corsons, the pet dogs "offered the residents of the nursing home a form of non-threatening, reassuring, nonverbal communication and tactile comfort and thus helped break the vicious cycle of loneliness, hopelessness and social withdrawal." One resident, who for twenty-six years had been totally withdrawn, reentered the social environment of the nursing home after introduction to a pet dog. A major conclusion of the Corsons was that companion animals acted as an effective socializing catalyst for the residents.

Mugford and McComiskey examined the placement of parakeets in homes of the elderly in England.(5) Robb has quantified behavior characteristics of elderly males in a VA hospital in Pittsburgh through the placement of a puppy in the activity room of the hospital.(6) A survey of staff members of a geriatric ward of a hospital conducted by Brickel found that companion animals on the ward promoted patient responsiveness.(7) It also provided patients additional opportunities to give as well as receive affection. These studies support the conclusion of the Corsons that companion animals may serve as a "social lubricant for humans."

The only known physiological parameters that have been extensively analyzed in the human-companion animal bond have been in the cardiovascular area. Lynch and other researchers have performed studies to assess the effect of social stimuli on the heart rate of humans and animals when they are in the presence of each other.(8) (9) (10) (11) Thomas et al. demonstrated a marked difference in heart rates of stable and nervous dogs when petted by a human.(12) The nervous dogs showed no change while the normal dogs showed a marked decrease. Friedmann et al. reported a significant difference in survival rates of coronary care patients who owned companion animals compared to those who did not own animals.(13) Of thirty-nine patients who did not own animals, eleven died within a year of discharge while only three of fifty-three companion-animal-owning patients died during the same time period. One must question if this difference was due to the benefits of animal ownership or rather due to the psychosocial differences between people who are more likely to own animals compared to those who do not own animals.

The literature has espoused the concerns as well as the benefits in the utilization of animals in health care facilities. Disadvantages described by various authors include the physical harm that the animal may cause to the resident, zoonotic diseases (diseases transmitted to humans by animals), lack of proper facilities for the animals, improper sanitation, allergies of the residents and staff to the animals, expense of the animals and skepticism of any possible therapeutic value of animals to human behavior. To assess the degree of these possibilities, several studies were initiated at the University of Minnesota.

A SURVEY OF 762 LONG-TERM CARE FACILITIES

When the Minnesota legislature passed a law in February, 1979, stating, "Nursing homes may keep pet animals on the premises subject to reasonable rules as to the care, type and maintenance of the pet," numerous questions arose. "What are appropriate guidelines for allowing animals in health care institutions? What constitutes a "good" companion animal program? What are the actual advantages and disadvantages of allowing companion animals in these facilities?

To seek answers to these questions, the University of Minnesota Center to Study Human-Animal Relationships and Environments surveyed nursing homes, supervised living facilities, boarding care homes and hospital attached nursing homes through a mailed questionnaire. Nearly 50 percent of all Minnesota health care facilities reported that they were currently utilizing companion animals.

Four types of animal programs were noted; (1) non-scheduled visiting animal, (2) scheduled visiting animal, (3) resident animal and (4) facilitated therapy animal programs. A non-scheduled visiting animal program allows for family members and/or friends of the health care facility resident to bring a companion animal to visit the resident. This animal may be the resident's animal which had to be "given up" on admission to the facility. These visits are considered non-scheduled as there is no formal animal visiting program. In this case, the companion animal comes with the family or friend when they visit the resident. Conversely, a scheduled visiting animal program entails companion animals being brought to a health care facility on an appointment or regular interval basis. Organizations such as humane societies, 4-H clubs and even the city zoo may schedule animal visiting programs. These programs provide an entertainment format for residents, and actual one-to-one human-animal contact may be minimal.

Resident animal programs include animals owned and cared for by an individual resident or animals that are considered mascots of the facility and are therefore owned and cared for by the facility. The term animal-facilitated therapy has a broad range of meanings. It may refer to the above programs or a structured form of therapy where a therapist, as an adjunct to treatment of a physical or emotional condition, uses a companion animal to bridge the environment with a withdrawn resident.

There was little variation among responses of administrators by type of health care facility. However, administrators who utilize animal programs identified many more advantages than disadvantages of their programs, while administrators who do not utilize animal programs perceived many more disadvantages than advantages.

The administrators stated that maintaining proper sanitation and hygiene was their greatest concern, but rarely did an administrator state that an animal had been removed because of sanitation problems. While animal programs were perceived to be beneficial, the nursing home did not want the extra work of maintaining a resident animal program. Reluctance of staff to take on extra work and/or the lack of acceptance by staff and residents to the companion animals were also viewed as disadvantages. Liability of the health care facility for possible injuries caused by residents tripping over small dogs or cats was considered a potential problem by some. Administrators of many supervised living facilities for the mentally retarded were more concerned about the potential abuse an animal might receive from a resident, something that occasionally occurs with the elderly also. Many administrators considered the three major dimensions of animal programs, namely, the overall welfare of staff, residents and animals.

Three of every four of the Minnesota facilities utilized dogs on the premises. Cats, fish and pet birds were the next most utilized animals. One of seven health care facilities had utilized either baby or adult farm animals in their animal programs. This is important as a sizeable proportion of elderly residents in nursing homes are from rural backgrounds. Reexposing elderly rural residents to farm animals may substantially rekindle pleasant memories of their past. The overall conclusion is that all domestic species of animals as well as many non-domestic species of animals were successful.

The animals provided entertainment and variety and were viewed as a positive mental stimulus in the environment. The animal not only gives affection but it also allows the resident to give affection. This point is very important, as the elderly tend to be more recipients than "givers" of love because opportunities for hugging or sexual relations are so limited. A companion animal allows the elderly socially acceptable affection.

RISK ASSESSMENT STUDIES

Anderson (16) studied the laws and regulations regarding pets in nursing homes in all 50 states. Half of the states have no prohibition of pets except that they are not allowed in food preparation areas or dining rooms. Sixteen states have specific legislation allowing pets. The other

9 states either prohibit all animals or limit the allowable types. There was no difference in pet related problems in states that regulated animals and those that didn't. Parenthetically, no owner or manager of federally assisted rental housing may prohibit or prevent a resident from having a household pet. (P.L. 98-181, 1983).

Beall, Greco, Anderson and Stryker (17) conducted a study of risks of allergies, infections and injuries from both visiting and live-in pets in 284 Minnesota nursing homes for one year (1984–85). Every home was surveyed monthly and exposure rates and incident rates were determined.

There were a total of 19 injuries in 18 homes during the year. Eight incidents were caused by mature pets, eight by puppies or kittens and three by outdoor animals. Two were serious (one broken shoulder and one broken wrist) and both occurred while a policy was violated. The other 17 injuries mainly consisted of minor scratches by kittens or puppies. There were no pet related incidents of any kind in the other 264 homes during the same year. The risk calculations were very low; for a serious injury — .18/1,000,000 person-hours of exposure time and for total animal incidents — 1.6/1,000,000 person-hours of exposure time. This compares to 526/1,000,000 person-hours from all non-animal related incidents unrelated to animals. The incidence rate for live-in animals was nearly identical to the rate for visiting animals that came from families, humane societies, volunteers and employees. There were no pet related infections or allergies.

Other types of reported incidents were examined in six of the homes reporting pet incidents. For every 1,000 incidents reported in these nursing homes, 4.5 were pet related and 995.5 were not related to pets. As one person observed, "pets seem to be safer than people."

COMPANION ANIMALS—YES OR NO?

People who work and live in a nursing home mirror the different feelings and perceptions of the general population toward animals. Some individuals do not like animals. Others may like dogs but dislike cats. Still others may actually be fearful of a particular species of animal. Others love all animals and still others are neutral in their feelings.

These varying perceptions and feelings about animals are especially significant in long-term care facilities that use animals to achieve specific therapeutic outcomes. These complex psychological factors have consequences for the outcome of the program. Design and operation of programs which will achieve therapeutic outcomes requires that both psychological and functional factors be addressed.

To do this, a "pre-program" survey designed to identify and examine all factors bearing on the operation of a proposed program is recommended. Based on the survey, an animal use program can be designed for the unique circumstances of a particular facility or a justifiable decision might be to not have an animal program.

Prior to conducting a preprogram survey, a knowledgeable animal use advocate might present the rationale of using animals as therapeutic adjuncts in long-term care to administrators and staff. At this time, the concept of various animal-facilitated therapy programs can be explained and the purpose of a preprogram survey established. Besides laying the foundation for the survey, this meeting can serve to make clear that any subsequent program will involve participation of both administration and staff for implementation.

In addition, monitoring and evaluation of benefits and costs is necessary. For example, in one nursing home, a resident cat that was dearly loved by the residents severely injured her paw in an automatic door. When brought to a veterinarian for treatment, it was found that no financial provisions had been made for veterinary care, and as a result, the cat was euthanized.

It is desirable to have the individual who will be responsible for the operation of a proposed program conduct the survey. This person will then become familiar with all aspects of the program under consideration and is better prepared to deal with situations and problems that will arise. The example of the injured nursing home cat illustrates such a situation. An outline of operation of the proposed program should be prepared.

Attitudinal Factors

The presence of animals in a health care facility, whatever their intended purpose, can be perceived in very different ways by individual administrators and staff. Understandably, personnel are concerned about any adverse effect on the environment and any additional or unwanted duties involved in caring for animals. These concerns are legitimate and must be addressed if an animal-use program is to succeed. In some cases, these concerns are complicated by individual feelings about animals in general, or a species of animal in particular.

These feelings need to be identified. Certainly if an administrator or key staff member does not want an animal program, success will be difficult. In such a situation, if all aspects of a proposed program are discussed and concerns are addressed, the program usually can be implemented on a trial basis. Then as the program develops, resolution of concerns can be evaluated.

As with administrators and staff, residents will vary in attitudes about animals. Persons who are allergic to animals or fear the animals need to be identified. Experience has shown that most long-term care residents seem to enjoy reminiscing about animals and especially about companion animals that they have had in the past. With some residents, questioning of relatives or friends to obtain this information may be necessary.

It has been helpful to use carefully selected visiting animals as a "social lubricant" to determine responses. During the survey, the idea of using animals in a structured program should be presented and discussed with the resident council. It is suggested that terms such as "pet therapy" be avoided and the concept of companionship and care of animals be emphasized. It is important that residents understand how they will be involved with the animals.

Operational Factors

Operational factors, in contrast to attitudinal factors, refer to functional realities such as environmental sanitation; animal disease and behavior concerns; selection, care and handling of animals, etc. It is emphasized, however, that attitudinal factors greatly affect these operational factors. For example, the act of defecation by a dog in a living area is viewed and handled very differently by a person who does not like dogs than by a person who loves dogs. Operational factors need attention **prior** to program start-up.

Suitability of Building and Grounds

While any long-term care facility building is probably suitable for visiting animal programs, it may not be so for other kinds of animal programs. A high-rise building in an urban area with no yard or grounds would not be suitable for a large resident dog. On the other hand, such a facility might be suitable for a resident cat. For any program, the building and premises must be considered in terms of the mechanics of caring for and managing animals.

Environmental Considerations

Animals may defecate, urinate, or shed hair and dandruff in inappropriate places. Besides this, some species can be noisy or difficult to train. Behavioral characteristics of animals should be consistent with the environment. Experience has indicated, however, that these environmental occurrences are infrequent, and not difficult to handle. For example, the occasional "accident" by a visiting dog is usually promptly cleaned up by an embarrassed owner or handler, especially if paper towels, a receptacle for waste, and a mop and pail of sanitizing solution are readily available. The point is that recognizing that such "accidents" do happen and providing a means of dealing with the situation can eliminate the problem.

Animal Health

Consideration of factors bearing on the health of animals in a health-care facility involves two aspects: (1) the well-being of the animals, and (2) the prevention of exposure of residents and staff to animal diseases, especially animal diseases transmittable to man (zoonoses) and animal-caused injuries. Both require input and recommendations from a veterinarian. It is important that this veterinary involvement be included in the preplanning survey as a first step in preparing detailed procedures necessary to assure that animal programs are in compliance with accepted animal health requirements. Regulatory and licensing agencies will be especially concerned with this aspect of animal use programs. Prerequisites for animals to be used in resident or facilitated therapy programs include: 1) a health examination by a veterinarian to certify that the animal is free from signs of infectious diseases and 2) evidence of immunization against rabies (for dogs, cats, and other domestic animals such as horses) and other recommended immunizations.

To maintain health and well-being of resident animals, arrangements must be made for daily care such as feeding, shelter, grooming, training and exercise. The animals' living area must be cleaned and cared for. Arrangements for treatment of injuries and illness must be planned in addition to a continuing veterinary preventive medicine program of health examinations and periodic immunizations.

Animal Behaviors

The behavior of animals plays a key role in all animal programs. Unfortunately, animal behavior often becomes a factor after introduction of the animal. Criteria and procedures designed to evaluate behavior of animals at least for live-in programs will help to reduce this risk.

It has been found helpful in selecting suitable puppies, to include a puppy temperament test as part of the required health examination by a veterinarian. Such a behavioral examination, while not definitive, probably will identify animals with obvious inappropriate behavioral characteristics.

However, a preentrance health and temperament examination is not practical for visiting animals. These animals are usually family pets and exposure to residents is relatively brief. The facility can impose restrictions and rules for visiting animals to minimize animal diseases and injury risks. However, such procedures for handling situations of inappropriate visiting animal behavior (and perhaps the animal owner or handler) are necessary in advance of any incident.

To control visiting animals, a common procedure is to inform owners or handlers of visiting pets, in writing, of pet visiting requirements and rules, and indicate that the owner or handler is responsible for pet behavior during the visit. While this has been helpful, unless there are policies to handle violations of rules, problems may be handled inadequately.

Operational and Supervisory Factors

The functioning of every kind of animal program in a long-term care facility will involve administration and staff. It is helpful to construct an operational chart to identify areas and functions of facility participants. Who will participate in selecting the animal, writing policies and evaluating the program? Who will be responsible for the daily care of a resident animal or coordinating visiting programs?

SUMMARY

Based on mostly anecdotal evidence, various animal programs in long-term care facilities do contribute significantly to the health and well-being of residents. Unfortunately, at the present time, methods to quantify the advantages, and conversely, the disadvantages of a particular program are lacking. However, thorough planning will help administrators and staff to make judgments as to relative benefits and costs of a particular program. Monitoring and evaluation functions will provide answers for each facility. The authors believe that appropriate planning by a health care administrator will greatly enhance the potential benefits that can be obtained by residents and staff through the utilization of animals in a long-term health care facility.

RESOURCE

Lee, Ronnal et al. *Animals in Nursing Homes: Guidelines.* California Veterinary Medical Association (order File No. 3758, P.O. Box 60,000, San Francisco, CA 94160), 1987 or from the Delta Society, Century Building, Suite 303, 321 Burnett Ave., South, Renton, WA 98055.

REFERENCES

1. Bustad, L. K. The contributions of companion animals to human well being. *Animals, Aging and the Aged,* Minneapolis, University of Minnesota Press 1980.
2. Levinson, B. *Pets and Human Development.* Springfield, IL, Charles C Thomas, Publisher, 1972.
3. Corson, S. A., and Corson, E. D. Pets as mediators of therapy. *Current Psychiatric Therapies 18:*195–205, 1978.
4. Corson, S. A., and Corson, E. D., Gwynne, P. H. Pet facilitated psychotherapy. In Anderson R. S. (ed.) *Pet Animals and Society.* Springfield, IL, Charles C Thomas, Publisher, 1975.
5. Mugford, R. A., and McComiskey, J. G. Some recent work on the psychotherapeutic value of caged birds with older people. In Anderson, R. S. (ed.) *Pet Animals and Society.* Springfield, IL, Charles C Thomas, Publisher, 1975.
6. Robb, S. S., Boyd, M., and Pristash, C. L. A wine bottle, plant and a puppy. *Journal of Gerontological Nursing 6(12):*721–728, 1980.
7. Brickel, C. M. The therapeutic role of cat mascots with a hospital-based geriatric population. A staff survey. *Gerontologist 19:*368–372, 1979.
8. Lynch, J. J. et al. The effects of human contact on cardiac arrhythmia in coronary care patients. *J Nerv Ment Dis 158:*88–98, 1974.
9. Lynch, J. J. et al. Human contact and cardiac arrhythmia in a coronary care unit. *Psychosom Med 39:*183–188, 1977.
10. Lynch, J. J., McCarthy, J. F. The effect of petting on a classically conditioned emotional response. *Behav Res Ther 5:*55–62, 1967.
11. Lynch, J. J., Fregin, G. F., Mackie, J. B., and Monroe, R. R. The effect of human contact on the heart activity of the horse. *Psychophysiol 11:*472–478, 1974.
12. Thomas, K. J., Murphree, O. D., Newton, J. E. The effect of person on nervous and stable pointer dogs. *Conditional Reflex 5:*74–81, 1972.
13. Friedmann, E., Katcher, A., Lynch, J. J., and Thomas, S. A. Animal companions and one-year survival of patients after discharge from a coronary care unit. *Public Health Reports 95(4):*307–312, 1980.
14. Minnesota State Board of Health Rules and Regulations for Construction, Maintenance, Operation and License of Nursing Homes and Boarding Care Homes. Minneapolis, Minnesota Department of Health.

15. Minnesota State Board of Health Rules and Regulations for Construction, Maintenance, Operation and License of Supervised Living Facilities. Minneapolis, Minnesota Department of Health.

16. Anderson, R. K. et al Ed. *The Pet Connection: It's Influence on Our Health and Quality of Life.* South St. Paul, MN, Globe publishing, pp. 372–380, 1984.

17. Beale, N. et al, *Pet Related Risks in Nursing Homes,* unpublished MPH thesis, University of Minnesota 1986.

Chapter 22

CARE OF THE DYING AMONG FRIENDS

PETER W. THOREEN AND RUTH STRYKER

AN OVERVIEW OF PRACTICES

While one often reads that only 4 or 5 percent of those over sixty-five reside in nursing homes at any one time, over twenty percent of all deaths occur in nursing homes. Kastenbaum and Candy have labelled this the "4 percent fallacy." This statistic makes it evident that a long-term care administrator plays a major role in seeing that dying residents receive appropriate care in a supportive environment.

A review of the now voluminous literature on death and dying reveals very little attention to the specific problems of long-term care facilities. The literature does document that in general, the aged, including those in long-term care facilities, are less fearful and more accepting of death than the rest of American society. But much of the literature is biased toward the hospital and its problems in dealing with death and dying. Although much nursing literature is geared toward the dying patient, the reader is often left to interpret its applicability to the long-term care setting.

Because approximately 90 percent of the direct care delivered in long-term care settings (Vladeck, p. 19) is given by a nursing assistant, training in this area becomes an issue. While some states may require at least minimum training of nursing assistants, there is no guarantee that they are at all prepared to provide care and support to the dying. Also, no one has appeared to study and assess the quality or effect of inservice and orientation training programs on death and dying in long-term care facilities. One author's research concluded (although finding few statistically significant results) that working in nursing homes actually leads to **further avoidance** of death by the generally young and inexperienced nursing assistant (Howard).

A number of authors have examined how individual long-term care facilities, as "communities" and social institutions, have dealt with and affected the handling of death and dying (Gubrium, Marshall, Koff, 1975). According to Marshall: "administrative practices mitigate against interaction so as to create the conditions for death to be faced without community support" (p. 365). Koff stresses that the administrator needs to pay attention to policies and practices that support dealing with death as a natural part of life and openly recognize the psychosocial needs of the dying. Unfortunately, the literature offers administrators few concrete suggestions to improve care of the terminally ill resident. In a recent summary of research on attitudes toward death in the long-term care facility, Haber et al., made the following statement:

> Despite the frequency of death, few institutional administrators have given much thought to the special problems of the dying, nor have researchers given much attention to the effects of dying and death on residents and staff in long term care institutions (p. 25).

Hospice care is a philosophy or approach to care by attempting to address the total care needs of the terminally ill and their families. Healy's excellent article entitled "Hospice—What is It?" will serve to identify some key elements of hospice care:

- treatment of the patient and family together as a unit of care;
- service availability to patients on a home care and inpatient basis; twenty-four hours a day, seven days a week, with emphasis on medical and nursing skills;
- care at home is the goal and priority;
- interdisciplinary care team;
- physician directed services;
- central administration and coordination of services, use of volunteers;
- acceptance to the program based on health needs, not ability to pay;
- bereavement follow-up service to family.

Healy also explains as follows:

> These elements, which may be found in different combinations and concentrations, constitute a philosophy of care more than the foundation of a specific program. The key to hospice is continuity in the coordination of services. This one consideration tends to place hospice outside the current U. S. health care system, where acute care and long term care tend to be discrete processes (p. 51).

This is an important point. The administrator should realize that hospice may refer to a "philosophy" of care, a "program" of care, or a "place" where care is given. One can embrace and practice the **philosophy** of care, implement a full-fledged hospice **program**, or devote beds to the delivery of inpatient hospice care (**place**).

The literature often claims that "hospice care" can be delivered in any setting. This is true, but most hospice programs with designated inpatient beds are at acute care hospitals where a high number of nursing hours needed by terminal patients translates to staffing ratios not generally feasible (for reimbursement reasons) in long-term care facilities. Therefore, financing the staffing levels needed to meet the needs of multiple terminal residents and their families becomes a major stumbling block to a hospice program in long-term care facilities. In addition to the financial issues, potential problems include: training staff, providing a continuity of service, obtaining adequate physician involvement and support, and justifying the additional attention and services for the terminal resident as opposed to others.

Undoubtedly, many long-term care facilities have implemented, or are attempting to implement, components of the hospice philosophy of care. But it is questionable, to say the least, whether most facilities will be able to or should carry out full service hospice programs.

A STUDY OF MINNESOTA LONG–TERM CARE FACILITIES

In 1981, the Minnesota Coalition For Terminal Care, a non-profit organization concerned with improving care of the terminally ill, surveyed a random sample of Minnesota nursing homes to determine needs and practices related to dying residents. Of the 118 homes surveyed, eighty-nine (75%) responded. Most respondents were either Directors or Assistant Directors of Nursing.

There were a total of 1,820 deaths at the eighty-nine facilities during the study year, with an average of twenty-one per facility. Of these deaths, approximately 60 percent of the deaths were anticipated by staff. One of the criteria of admittance to most hospice programs is a diagnosis of terminal illness with a prognosis of six months or less to live. Only 5 percent of the responding facilities **did not** accept terminally ill residents, and all but one respondent agreed that there were particular and unique care needs associated with the terminally ill.

Some Needs Identified

The following summarizes the responses to specific questions:

What are the special needs of dying patients?

- special physical care needed (48%)
- dynamics of family involvement (55%)
- emotional care of resident (76%)
- spiritual needs of resident (36%)
- support of staff and other residents (15%)

What concerns you most when a resident becomes terminally ill?

Type of Response/Concern	No. %
• Meeting of spiritual and emotional needs	22 (25%)
• Meeting family needs	24 (25%)
• Making resident comfortable	32 (36%)
• Open communication with resident and family	19 (21%)
• Having sufficient and well trained staff	20 (23%)
• No answer	4 (5%)

The responses clearly indicate that the respondents were concerned about addressing the psychosocial needs of the resident **and** family, along with the physical comfort of the resident.

What problems have you most often observed with direct care-givers (staff nurses and aides) when a resident becomes terminally ill?

Problem	No. %
• Staff avoidance	59 (66%)
• Communication problems	65 (73%)
• Difficulty with accepting their own feelings	59 (66%)
• Giving supportive care	76 (85%)
• General discomfort	67 (75%)
• No answer	7 (8%)

What materials on specific topics for in-service education programs are needed? The top six answers were as follows.

Subject Area	# Checked	(% of 89)	Rank
Comfort care for the dying	56	63%	1
Talking about death with family members	55	62%	2
Talking about death with residents	54	61%	3
How to handle a family's grief	53	60%	4
Understanding one's own grief	51	57%	5
Care in the last 24 hours of life	49	55%	6

Respondents were asked: "What care practices are followed in your facility **after** a resident has died?"

Type of Practice	No. %)
Body Preparation	51 (57%)
Routine Notifications	52 (58%)
Attention to Needs of Staff & Residents	45 (51%)
Family Support	46 (52%)
No answer	2 (2%)

Very few respondents actually indicated that specific policies or procedures existed to deal with death and care of the dying. There were strong feelings expressed about isolating or not isolating the body after death. Interestingly, a fair number of facilities mentioned that they not only encouraged other residents to attend the funeral or visitation, but also provided transportation to do so.

How many hours are devoted to in-service education on terminal care in a year?

Category of Hours	No. %
none	4 (4%)
1	9 (10%)
1–2	27 (30%)
3–4	29 (33%)
5–6	7 (8%)
7–8	0 (0%)
9–10	2 (2%)
12	9 (10%)
No Answer	2 (2%)

While almost all respondents accepted terminal residents and indicated that they felt they had unique needs, 45 percent indicated they only offered two or fewer in-service hours a year on this topic. Eighty-three percent mentioned that only nursing staff attended training sessions and 49 percent indicated that all staff were encouraged to attend. The latter, sensitizing **all** staff to the needs of the dying and their families, is stressed in the literature.

Are there specific state or federal policies that inhibit your ability to provide appropriate care and services to terminally ill residents? Sixty-nine percent of the respondents answered "no" to this question. Of those who responded "yes" (27%), most mentioned the limited reimbursement available for additional nursing staff. The majority of facilities did feel that public policies **were not** a major stumbling block in providing better care to the terminally ill.

DYING AMONG FRIENDS: THE LONG-TERM CARE ADMINISTRATOR'S ROLE AND CHALLENGE

This section will focus on the administrator's role in improving the care and support of dying residents and their families. First, it is important to reflect briefly on what goals and objectives are to be achieved. It must be recognized that the expected outcome is death, and it will almost always be an emotional and difficult time for all involved. Therefore, the administrator must focus on goals surrounding death, such as allowing each resident to die a **dignified death** and providing a setting where family, staff and other residents can at least have the opportunity to grow and learn from the dying and death they experience. The administrator should also remember that what constitutes a "dignified death" will ultimately be defined by each resident and family unit. However, the organization must lay the ground for a "dignified death" through such care objectives as: maintaining the resident pain-free, by providing supportive care that preserves "comfort, hygiene and dignity" rather than prolongs life; facilitating quality family involvement and interaction if appropriate; allowing the dying person to maintain control of decisions; and by providing support to staff, other residents and family.

Organizational Philosophy

As with all services and programs of the long-term care facility, those aimed at care of the dying should be related to the organization's overall philosophy. If this cannot be done, it may not be appropriate for the facility to care for the dying at all. In such cases, the goal or objective should probably be to discharge care of the resident to the appropriate provider. For example, if an intermediate care facility's stated philosophy of care is "to provide quality residential services to persons needing minimum nursing and support services," it may not be appropriate to provide end-stage, terminal care to residents needing heavy nursing care. On the other hand, if the stated philosophy of a facility offering multiple levels of nursing care is "to provide quality services to all residents where medically feasible," this should allow the administrator to go ahead and develop appropriate goals and objectives to care for the dying resident.

Service Objectives and Goals

First, it will be important to think through the objectives and goals pertaining to services for the dying when the expected outcome is death. A facility may have the goal of: "restoring or maintaining each resident at the most independent level feasible." Is such a goal appropriate for the dying? It may be, but others such as the following may be more helpful:

- "provide a supportive and accepting environment where death and dying can be discussed openly;"
- "where medically feasible and desired, allow all residents to die with dignity without transfer out of the facility;"
- "work closely with other community providers to maximize support and services available to each dying resident and the family."

Goals and objectives can also serve as a focal point for evaluating the outcomes later. Next, the administrator should evaluate and list the specific needs and issues that will form the basis for practices, policies and protocols. This will help department heads to prioritize their efforts, and it again serves as an aid in evaluating progress at some later date.

Resident and Family Needs:

- The need for physical pain control measures;
- The need for focus on psychosocial concerns of resident and family;
- The need for privacy;
- The need for resident and family to deal with their grief;
- The need for resident and/or family to take care of "unfinished business";
- The need for continuity of care when energy is being drained by the dying process;
- The need to address spiritual concerns.

Staff Needs:

- The need for management to support and recognize the grief that staff may experience;
- The need to discuss what may be a young person's first death experience;
- The need to spend extra time with the terminal resident who has special physical, spiritual, and psychological needs;
- The need to get proper education and preparation on caring for the terminally ill.

Other Residents' Needs:

- The need for other residents to resolve their grief over the death of a significant friend in the facility;

- The need for other residents to feel secure that the staff and facility will help them die a dignified death;
- The need for other residents to help and support fellow residents in their dying;
- The need for residents to be informed of deaths occurring in the facility.

Policies and Practices

Supportive Care Guidelines

Limiting treatment is of course an antithesis to the basic values and education of health care professionals, especially physicians and nurses. However, the development of technology makes it mandatory that health care professionals think through responsible and appropriate applications of its capabilities. Some nursing home residents prefer that their health care be limited to preserving their comfort and dignity rather than prolonging life.

To achieve this goal, nursing homes must develop policies that will assure a medically responsible and ethical decision making process to protect the rights of residents and families. The guiding principle is to assure, whenever possible, that it is the resident who makes the final decision regarding withdrawal, withholding, continuance and initiation of treatment. The physician's role is to explain medical considerations and the consequences of various decision options. The role of staff is to encourage discussion of options and help to assure understanding the options. It is inappropriate for staff to give a personal opinion or judgment about any option.

A supportive care plan can be initiated by a resident, family member (or guardian), or physician, and should be initiated prior to a crisis event whenever possible. It is suggested that a care conference be arranged with the resident (regardless of competency), family, physician, a clergyman, and a representative from the nursing staff.

If a resident's competency is questionable and there is no designated representative, the health care team is obliged to determine their best judgment of what the resident would have wanted as a competent person. Information sources would include the resident, any previously written statements by the resident, the knowledge of family members, friends and others.

A supportive care plan may include such elements as 1) DNR—

withholding cardiopulmonary resusitation. This does not preclude assistance in the event of choking, shock, hemorrhage, etc. 2) DNI—withholding
endotracheal intubation in the event of respiratory failure, 3) avoid
hospitalization—a preference for care at home or in the nursing home
(except in the event of fracture, uncontrollable bleeding, or uncontrollable pain). 4) The name of the designated representative if the resident
is unable to make decisions, and 5) A list of any treatments that may be
unacceptable when restoration to health is impossible and extension of
life is of secondary importance.

A physician writes the orders for the supportive care plan and it must
be communicated to ALL staff. A plan might include comfort measures
such as relief of pain, good hygiene, skin care, oral hygiene, range of
motion, oral and nasal suctioning, maintaining bowel and bladder function and giving food and fluids by mouth. It also ensures dignity and
respect including psychosocial support, privacy, opportunities to visit
with family, friends and clergy. The plan should be reviewed every two
months. Most supportive care policies require a physician's order for
oxygen therapy, nasogastric feedings, gastrostomy feedings, laboratory
tests and medications or special treatments.

It is critical to document 1) the resident's desires, 2) the basis for
determining competency (or for determining an incompetent person's
wishes), 3) the significant persons involved in making the decision
(including their relationship to the resident), and 4) the rationale used to
determine the supportive care orders.

The above suggestions have been brought together from a great variety of supportive care policies in nursing homes. To develop a policy for
a particular home, it is recommended that the home either appoint a
Biomedical Ethics Committee of its own or use one already established
in the community, possibly at the local hospital. Supportive care policies
are usually developed and approved by such a committee which can also
be a valuable resource for families, residents and staff.

Orientation and In-Service Programs

Both orientation and in-service programs should have adequate time
devoted to death, dying and care of the terminally ill. A one hour
presentation is generally not enough. In assisting the in-service director
and evaluating the efforts in this area, the administrator should keep in
mind the following:

- The facility must invest adequate time and money in educating staff on these topics.
- The hospice philosophy of care should be taught and included in orientation programs.
- Staff should be allowed to discuss and share their own feelings about death and dying.
- The facility should make use of speakers and workshops offered in the community.

Family Involvement

Policies regarding family involvement in long-term care facilities should be an important part of the facility's policy manual. This is especially true when a resident is dying. The family should not only be allowed but encouraged to provide care whenever possible. The staff must not be "too busy" to pay attention to the needs and questions of family members.

Obviously, the pattern of family involvement with the long-term care facility may be set long before the resident approaches death. But the administrator should help staff remember that regardless of past involvement, families **may** feel a great need to be closer to the resident as death approaches due to feelings of genuine love and concern, guilt, or simply a desire to take care of "unfinished business" with their loved one.

The demands and needs of the dying are great. Families should be recognized as a resource to help meet these demands and needs, especially in light of realistic limits on staffing levels in long-term care facilities. Administrators must see that policies and procedures are in place that encourage family involvement.

If there is no available family, staff, friends and other residents may fill the family role for the resident. This, of course, suggests that "substitute" families may experience more intense grief and need support themselves.

Special Care Practices and Programs

The administrator should take the time to evaluate the feasibility and appropriateness of special care practices and programs for the dying. In doing this, the administrator needs to weigh the strengths and weaknesses of the organization and realistically assess the feasibility and importance of implementing such practices and programs. Some specific suggestions are:

1. **Development of a Hospice Program:**
   As mentioned earlier, this may or may not be feasible. At minimum, the administrator should look at what hospice principles can be applied at his/her facility and how the hospice philosophy of care should be integrated into existing practices. (See: **Standards of a Hospice Program of Care,** National Hospice Organization.)
2. **Developing an "Internal Specialist":**
   Training or hiring a staff nurse to specialize in care of the dying. This person would then manage the care of all dying residents.
3. **Support Groups for Families of Dying Residents:**
   This may be feasible for very large homes. It should be remembered that these groups are difficult to run and skilled facilitators are necessary. It may be more appropriate to refer families elsewhere if other community groups are available.
4. **Interdisciplinary Care Team With Volunteers:**
   Another idea is to pull together a special committee or team of staff members to discuss and coordinate the care of dying residents. Volunteers can be trained and used to assist staff and family in meeting needs of the dying.

It should be remembered that the dying need good physical care. Because hospice programs have developed expertise in the areas of pain control and symptom relief for the dying, area programs should be consulted for their expertise.

Attention to Physical Surroundings

In general, this should not be a major problem for long-term care facilities, as they are already more "homelike" than hospitals. The dying may wish to be surrounded by familiar and special objects which the staff should facilitate if possible. In addition, there may be a need for privacy with family. Since many residents share rooms with others, the administrator may wish to keep a private room available for special circumstances. It should be remembered that "roommates" may be a source of support and comfort. The dying should not be routinely isolated or moved from their own bed and room. Residents may specifically request not to be removed to a hospital so that they may die among their friends.

Residents as Care Givers

Fellow long-term care residents may be a great source of comfort and support to one another through the dying process. Staff should be made aware of this and help facilitate material support and kindness shown between residents. An administrator responding to the Minnesota study writes:

> The terminally ill need the comfort and encouragement from our other residents, and by the same token, they are facing their own deaths by teaching others how to die. I have seen our "up and about" residents sitting by the bedside of one who is dying—the relationships are beautiful.

When appropriate and when asked, staff should be honest in telling other residents that someone is dying and needs their support. The long-term care organization is no place for what is often referred to as the "conspiracy of silence."

Staff Support Mechanisms

It may be important to implement structured support mechanisms to help staff in dealing with their own grief over residents' deaths or simply to relieve some of the tension and stress that often surrounds care of the terminally ill.

It may be necessary to have some intentional ways to allow staff members to share, discuss and learn from their experiences and feelings. Some mechanisms to do this are as follows:

- Hold a regular support group for staff where they can share their feelings regarding the loss of a resident close to them. These may also provide a good forum to introduce ideas and suggestions as to how to handle and deal with future deaths as well as a time to simply receive some support and empathy from others.
- Use a "buddy system" and assign younger more inexperienced staff to more experienced staff who have a healthy outlook on death. After some training and encouragement, older staff may be able to assist and support their younger counterparts in dealing with death and dying. There should be structured, paid time for the two persons to share experiences when a dying resident is being cared for or has died.
- Have a structured "remembrance" session for the staff after a death has occurred. Possibly ask each staff member close to the person who died to share some thoughts, a poem, a reading, etc. about them. This could be included with a more formal memorial service and could also include the family.
- It is also a good idea to have a consulting psychiatrist, psychologist or psychiatric social worker who can intervene and assist staff members who need more formal professional help.

In general, one of the best support "mechanisms" will be a strong orientation and in-service educational focus on death and dying that helps prepare staff for the issues surrounding care of the terminally ill. This, in combination with promoting an environment of open communications about death and dying, set by example of the administrator, will serve as a constant support system.

None of the mechanisms should be implemented overnight. They require trained professionals who are able to recognize pathological grief needing professional referral, and staff who are able to tap the natural support system a facility will have in its more experienced and caring staff members.

Links With Community Resources

One of the most important tasks is to examine the organization's links and relationships with community resources to assist in improving care of their dying residents. The administrator should establish working relationships with area hospice programs, grief support groups, home health agencies, the local cancer society, etc. An important aspect of care of the dying is continuity. A long-term care facility can be an important link between home and the hospital as the care needs of a terminally ill person change.

Many resources in the community may be able to assist with staff education needs in this area. Many hospice programs will do in-service programs for long-term care facilities free of charge. At minimum, the administrator with the help of the social worker should compile a list of resource capabilities and services. Without such resources, the facility will be unable to assure that dying residents and their families will receive the most appropriate and highest quality terminal care. The author knows a long-term care director of nursing who wrote to a well-known hospice program 1,500 miles away in search of better pain control methods for the dying, not knowing that over ten hospice programs existed in that person's home state.

Practices and Policies That Follow a Death

When asking long-term care administrators about practices and policies following a death, most will quickly refer the inquirer to the policy on "preparation of the body following death" and on "notification of relatives upon death" in the nursing policy manual. These policies are obviously necessary, but the administrator should also think about more meaningful practices and policies. Some suggestions are as follows:

- assisting staff and other residents in going to funerals held outside the facility;
- holding the funeral or memorial service in the facility; it is important to recognize the bereavement needs of other residents, to allow them to express their grief and to honor the memory of the deceased;
- do not attempt to hide the fact that a death has occurred; deal with it openly and in a forthright manner; if other residents ask about a person who has died, they should be given accurate information; this does not mean announcing the death over the loudspeaker, but it does mean allowing natural communications to work. One administrator suggests a more formal recognition of the death and life that was lived: "We have a flower and an easel with a typed sheet pertaining to the resident's life sitting by the front door until after the funeral. This seems to tell the other residents that we will remember them too when they die."
- the administrator should write a personal letter to each family following the death of a resident. In addition, the administrator should also encourage other staff who were close to the resident to do so.
- if the facility experiences deaths frequently and is fairly large, it may be feasible to think about a formal bereavement support group for families. Or the administrator may offer a meeting room at the facility for a community-based bereavement group to which families can be referred if the need arises. This is again something that requires trained professionals and should not be done without an accurate assessment of need and community alternatives. At minimum, someone in the facility should be attuned to recognizing pathological grief reactions in families in order to make the proper referrals.

The importance of such practices and policies after a death cannot be stressed enough. It is crucial that other relatives and their families know that death will be handled with dignity and that the lives that were lived will be honored and remembered with respect by staff and the long-term care facility overall.

In Summary: A Challenge

This chapter has attempted to provide the long-term care administrator with ideas for a Model (see Figure 22–1) to improving care of the dying resident and his/her family. The long-term care facility will continue to play an important role in caring for the dying, and the administrator has the responsibility of seeing that it is carried out appropriately and with sensitivity and commitment to quality.

In closing, the following "Dying Person's Bill of Rights" should be used as a challenge in attempting to implement some of the suggestions offered in this chapter.

The Dying Person's Bill of Rights*

I have the right to be treated as a living human being until I die.

I have the right to maintain a sense of hopefulness, however changing its focus may be.

I have the right to be cared for by those who can maintain a sense of hopefulness, however changing this might be.

I have the right to express my feelings and emotions and my approaching death, in my own way.

I have the right to participate in decisions concerning my care.

I have the right to expect continuing medical and nursing attention, even though "cure" goals must be changed to "comfort" goals.

I have the right not to die alone.

I have the right to be free from pain.

I have the right to have my questions answered honestly.

I have the right not to be deceived.

I have the right to have help from and for my family in accepting my death.

I have the right to die in peace and dignity.

I have the right to retain my individuality and not be judged for my decisions, which may be contrary to the beliefs of others.

I have the right to discuss and enlarge my religious and/or spiritual experiences, regardless of what they mean to others.

I have the right to expect that the sanctity of the human body will be respected after death.

I have the right to be cared for by caring, sensitive, knowledgeable people who will attempt to understand my needs and will be able to gain some satisfaction in helping me face my death.

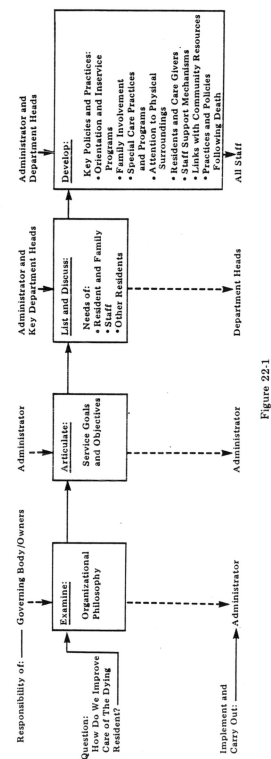

A Model Approach to Improving Care Of The Dying Long-Term Care Residents

Figure 22-1

REFERENCES

Dubois, Paul M. *The Hospice Way of Death.* New York, Human Sciences Press, 1980.

Gubrium, Jaber F. *Living and Dying at Murray Manor.* New York, St. Martin's Press, 1975.

Haber, David; Joanne Tuttle and Mary Rogers. Attitudes About Death in the Nursing Home: A Research Note, *Death Education,* 5, pp. 25–28, 1981.

Healy, William. Hospice . . . What is It?" *American Health Care Association Journal.* July 1980, pp. 51–56.

Howard, Elaine. The Effect of Work Experience in a Nursing Home on the Attitudes Toward Death Held by Nurses Aides, *Gerontologist,* 14(1), February 1974, pp. 54–56.

Ingram, Donald K. and John R. Barry. National Statistics on Deaths in Nursing Homes, *Gerontologist,* Vol. 17(4), 1977, pp. 303–308.

Kastenbaum, Robert and Sandra E. Candy. The 4% Fallacy: A Methodological and Empirical Critique of Extended Care Facility Population Statistics, *International Journal of Aging and Human Development,* Vol. 4(1), 1973, pp. 15–21.

Katz, Barry P.; Michael S. Zoeb and Gene D. Therriault. Where People Die, *Public Health Reports,* Vol. 94(6), Nov.–Dec., 1979, pp. 522–527.

Koff, Theodore H. Social Rehearsal for Death and Dying, *Journal of Long Term Care Administration,* 3(3), Summer, 1975, pp. 42–53.

Kramer, Jeannette R. Administrator Helps Determine the Quality of Dying, *Modern Nursing Home,* April 1970, pp. 49–52.

Lerner, Monroe. When, Why and Where People Die, in *The Dying Patient,* edited by Orville G. Brim, Jr., Howard E. Freeman, Sol Levine and Norman A. Scotch, New York, Russell Sage Foundation, 1970, pp. 5–29.

Marshall, Victor W. Organizational Features of Terminal Status Passage in Residential Facilities for the Aged, *Urban Life,* Vol. 4(3), Oct. 1975, pp. 349–368.

Minnesota State Department of Health. *Directory Licensed and Certified Health Care Facilities — 1980.* Minneapolis, Minnesota State Department of Health, 1980.

National Center for Health Statistics (NCHS). Discharges from Nursing Homes 1977 National Nursing Home Survey, Series 13, NCHS, U. S. Dept. of Health and Human Services, Hyattsville, MD, *preliminary unpublished report.*

National Center for Health Statistics (NCHS). *1977 — National Nursing Home Survey,* DHEW Pub. No. (PHS) 79-1794, U. S. DHEW, Public Health Service, Office of Health Research Statistics and Technology, NCAS, Hyattsville, MD, July 1979.

National Hospice Organization (NHO). *Standards of a Hospice Program of Care, 6th Revision,* Virginia, National Hospice Organization, February 23, 1979.

Thoreen, Peter W. *Death, Dying and Terminal Care: Issues Faced by the Long Term Care Facility,* Minneapolis, Coalition for Terminal Care, Inc., 1981.

Vladeck, Bruce C. *Unloving Care: The Nursing Home Tragedy.* New York, Basic Books, Inc., 1980.

Wershow, Harold J. The Four Percent Fallacy: Some Further Evidence and Policy Implications, *Gerontologist,* 16 (Vol. 1, Part 1), 1976, pp. 52–55.

PART VI

CREATING THE FUTURE

Every administrator is engaged in long-range planning which requires a well-informed vision of the next three to five years. The nursing home of 1965 was very different from the home of 1975 which was a world apart from those in 1985.

Evaluating one's organization and leading it successfully through altered political times and new scientific advances requires a thorough knowledge of how to measure present activities and an understanding of the change process and how to manage it. An eye to assuring quality and administrative skill in managing change allow an organization not only to weather turbulent times, but to create much of its own future. Chapter 23, Assuring Quality, and Chapter 24, Managing Change, address these increasingly important managerial skills.

Chapter 23

ASSURING QUALITY

Judy Eggleston

INTRODUCTION

This book has addressed the major aspects of quality long-term care. All of these aspects; an organizational direction guided by the mission statement, a skilled leader, competitive human resource management practices, and professional expertise must not only be in place, but the entire system must be under constant scrutiny. This is done through a quality assurance system which measures the quality of life of residents, not unlike regular systems used to monitor financial performance.

Today's administrator works in an environment of competition, knowledgable consumers, patient advocates, government regulations and ever-changing cost containment efforts. An understanding of the quality assurance process and a knowledge of how to apply its principles are fundamental to creative long-term care administration. This chapter provides an overview of the quality assurance process and its application to long-term care.

APPROACHES TO QUALITY

What do we mean by quality? The word expresses the relative worth of things, such as good quality vs. poor quality. Webster defines it as "the degree of excellence which a thing possesses." However, quality is intangible and difficult to define in long term care, as in most service industries. Residents, families, consumer advocates, health care professionals, regulators, the community and providers all have different ideas about what constitutes quality.

In 1984 Parasuraman, Zeithaml and Berry reported that researchers and managers of service firms concur that quality involves a comparison of performance with expectations. Expectations may range from simple adequacy to service unsurpassed by any other. Quality in long-term care is defined as CONFORMANCE TO EXPECTATIONS. While providers for the most part deliver quality based upon expectations, it must be measured and documented if we are assured of its quality. We must solicit expectations from our many publics, develop objective criteria, compare performance with expectations, make changes as needed, monitor the change, and document the results. Only then can we be sure we have quality! Quality assurance is therefore defined as an ongoing program which measures quality.

CONSUMER SATISFACTION

The primary consumer of long-term care services is the direct recipient of services. However, families, attending physicians, hospital discharge planners, social workers and others who influence resident placement are also consumers. This chapter will consider consumers collectively so that we look to the resident, consumer advocates and the health care community to give us definitions of quality.

One way consumers identify quality is to have staff who have a positive attitude toward residents (Spaulding). What is it then that staff must do and say to reflect a positive attitude? Residents, advocates, staff and published research/studies can identify specific staff behaviors which reflect a positive staff attitude. Examining each public's expectations provides the foundation for one set of quality measures.

PROFESSIONAL STANDARDS

The health care community defines the technical effectiveness of care and services. Individual practitioners, professional standards of practice and current research identify staff expectations.

Expectations are measured based upon resident outcomes and standardized procedures. Has the resident's medical condition improved or stabilized? Has the resident become more functionally independent? Has the resident been given the opportunities necessary to experience their optimal quality of life? It is critical to identify the expectations of each profession's quality criteria.

GOVERNMENT REGULATIONS

State and federal regulations provide baseline criteria for defining quality. The Health Care Financing Administration Conditions of Participation define fundamental compliance expectations for Medicaid and Medicare certification of long-term care facilities. Historically the regulations, implemented through the survey process, measured the CAPABILITY of the facility to deliver quality, NOT whether quality was provided. With the inception of the Long-Term Care Survey in 1986, the survey process better measures the quality provided to residents. The Health Care Financing Administration and state health departments define both compliance expectations and the evaluation process.

PLANNING FOR QUALITY

When quality is defined as conformance to the expectation of consumers, health care professionals and regulatory agencies, management has a basis for planning a quality assurance program. It requires making a commitment to quality by developing systems to assure that the quality of life provided residents is meeting expectations. Quality is enhanced by looking at yourself through the eyes of others.

The administrator and management team have the responsibility to develop the scope of the quality assurance program. It is based on the Mission Statement which reflects the values and commitments of the governing body to a·specific population of residents. Unique facility strengths such as religious affiliation or specialized services help to specify quality of life measures.

Human resource management practices are critical to the success of a quality assurance program. The right person to do the job, identification of performance expectations, tools for measuring employee performance and effective supervision are a critical base for providing quality care.

Management information systems provide important sources of data that can become a part of a quality assurance program. Reports of government surveys, grievances, complaint investigations, medical record audits, committee minutes and resident and family and employee surveys, provide valuable insights into current practice.

The overall responsibility and authority for the Quality Assurance Program rests with the administrator. However, the operation of the program is usually delegated to a Quality Assurance Committee. The committee should be interdisciplinary with representatives from every department, but not necessarily department heads. The committee chairperson, however, must be in a leadership position in order to direct the group toward facility-wide goals.

The committee should adopt a rewarding and non-threatening process. It should include ways to solicit and compile quality of care indicators from consumers, health care professionals, facility employees, and regulatory sources; mechanisms to use management information already compiled; systems to review, monitor and report compliance with regulatory agency standards; and a problem solving process to correct quality related problems with a built in system of follow-up.

THE QUALITY ASSURANCE PROCESS

ESTABLISHING GOALS

The first step to the quality assurance process is to establish goals. Goals must reflect the Mission Statement, organizational resources and industry trends. Perceptions of present quality should influence the goal direction.

Quality assurance goals may relate to structure, process or outcome.

STRUCTURE goals relate to organizational framework, physical environment and the kinds of human resources necessary to deliver care. They are the basics to quality—clean, safe environment and qualified staff. Structure goals are aligned with regulatory agency expectations.

PROCESS goals relate to HOW services and care are given. Does care comply with professional standards and/or facility procedures? For example, "residents will be assured prompt and comprehensive nursing and medical care" or "the Patient Bill of Rights will guide decision making."

OUTCOME goals reflect the status of the resident after care or service has been provided. Examples of outcome goals are "Ninety percent of the residents will state they are 'very satisfied' with meals" and "No more than five percent of residents will have an indwelling catheter." Concurrently, individual resident goals are developed through the care planning process. They are also critical to the quality assurance program.

DEFINING QUALITY INDICATORS

The second step in the quality assurance process is to define quality indicators. What do we see, hear and do to indicate that we are meeting facility goals and the expectations of our publics? For example, indicators for the goal, "Residents will be assured comprehensive medical and nursing care" might include 1) weight gains or losses in excess of 5 pounds will be reported to the physician and 2) the attending physician is notified immediately of any change in the resident's condition. Indicators of the goal, "Residents will be treated with respect" would include; 1) residents are dressed in their own clothing and are groomed daily, 2) staff speak to residents as adults and 3) staff knock before entering a resident's room.

Indicators are then organized into evaluation statements in order to be able to collect objective data which is the next step in the process.

COLLECTING DATA

There are four basic ways to gather data for measuring quality. They are documatation review, direct observation, survey, and interview.

DOCUMENTATION REVIEW is an audit of written documents. Both retrospective and concurrent review provide a picture of care given at a point in time. The most obvious is the medical record audit. Minutes of established committees, department head meetings, resident council meetings etc., should be reviewed for identification of problems and concerns, along with follow-up actions reported at later meetings.

DIRECT OBSERVATION is a report of care that is seen or heard. Observing the application of a sterile dressing with appropriate or inappropriate procedure is an example. Staff attitudes can be observed by the administrator, department head or a peer who sees or hears defined indicators such as staff greeting and helping visitors pleasantly, explaining procedures to residents and listening to a resident's expression of grief.

SURVEYS are written responses to a confidential questionnaire used to obtain feedback from consumers, staff or community members. The survey should enable respondents to rank their satisfaction and opinions and include open-ended questions to express real or perceived problems.

INTERVIEWS are structured one-on-one visits designed to elicit responses from individuals who may not answer written surveys. The interview can be conducted by facility personnel, but may be more effective when done by an objective third party. A data collection tool is necessary to document responses during or following an interview.

ANALYZING DATA

The fourth step in the quality assurance process is to review and analyze the data. Does actual performance equal expected performance as it is defined by an indicator? Whenever it does not, a decision must be made. IS THE PROBLEM RELATED TO FACILITY QUALITY? The problem may be one that requires attention to only one person's plan of care. IS IT PREVALENT? It may be so infrequent that it does not warrant a corrective action. CAN THE PROBLEM BE SOLVED? A service may not be offered because it simply is not available in a particular community.

If the committee decides to take no action, the reasons should be communicated to the group who identified the problem. If the problem requires further study and action, it is returned to the full process.

CORRECTIVE ACTION

When there is a difference between performance and expectations, a corrective action must be planned and implemented. Corrective action is determined by the apparent cause of the problem. Is there a lack of knowledge on the part of care givers? If so, would a change in hiring practices, better orientation, staff development or improved facility communications be helpful? Is there inappropriate behavior on the part of an individual or group? The corrective action may require improved supervisory practices. Or does the problem require a systems change?

Corrective actions must be thought of as constructive, not punitive. The next chapter on Change should be read carefully before embarking on major practice changes.

MONITORING THE PROCESS

Monitoring, the sixth step of the quality assurance process, either provides verification that the problem no longer exists and remains resolved or indicates that it needs greater attention. On-going review of performance against predetermined indicators and self-monitoring by employees are the keys to maintaining an effective program. Staff can be proud in knowing that their organization both identifies and maintains quality standards.

REEVALUATING GOALS

The final step of a quality assurance program is to reevaluate goals so that the process perpetuates itself as an integral part of the organizational culture. If a corrective action does not result in goal attainment, indicators may need to be redefined or the action may have to be reconsidered. When goals are attained, new expectations from various sources will need to be incorporated into the system. A good quality assurance process helps to maintain a creative atmosphere.

CONCLUSION

The long-term care administrator is responsible for providing assurances that the lives of residents meet both expectations and recognized standards of care. The quality assurance program must not only identify and correct problems but it must identify areas that can be enhanced and done better. In addition, it must identify accomplishments.

Quality is everyone's responsibility, but for the most part, quality is in the hands of direct care staff. They must be committed to quality assurance activities and receive appropriate recognition of their efforts if the program is to be successful. On-going feedback through an established communications network for staff, consumers and the community is essential to keep the process going.

With a creative and participative approach, the system will continually improve, as measured by regulatory agency compliance, technical and professional growth of staff and most significantly, resident/consumer satisfaction.

REFERENCES

American Health Care Association Journal. "Measuring Quality Care." July, 1985.

Beverly Enterprises. *Beverly Enterprises Quality Assurance Program.* January, 1984.

Kugler, Deborah; Nash, Trudy B.; Weinberger, Gail E. Quality Assurance: The Monitoring Process. *Contemporary Administrator.* February, 1984.

Parasuraman, A.; Zeithaml, Valarie A.; Berry, Leonard L. *A Conceptual Model of Service Quality and Its Implications for Future Research.* Texas A & M University. August, 1984.

Spaulding, Joy, Ph.D. *A Consumer Perspective on Quality Care: The Residents' Point of View.* A Project of the National Citizens' Coalition for Nursing Home Reform. February, 1985.

Chapter 24

MANAGING CHANGE

RUTH STRYKER AND GEORGE KENNETH GORDON

Administrative skill in managing change enables an organization to weather turbulent times and to create much of its own future. This skill is developed through understanding the nature of change, various concepts of change, ways to support people during the change process and the application of specific well-timed administrative interventions.

Long-term care administrators pursuing graduate studies at the University of Minnesota are introduced to systematic mastery of change theories, strategies and processes. In addition, they are required to initiate and conduct as well as document outcomes of a planned change project in their own organizations. These projects continue to reveal the susceptibility to deadly routinization of the daily round of activities and demonstrate the need for adept leadership by the administrator to cultivate and maintain the nursing home's capacity for progress.

THE NATURE OF CHANGE

Change is a dynamic process of transition, alteration and becoming different. It is not the goal (that was determined in the planning process), it is the "getting there"; it is the trip, if you will, rather than the destination. The trip may be good or bad. Indeed, the same change may be perceived as good by one individual or group and bad by another, so that reactions to change can be expected to vary among individuals and departments. Change is a part of our daily lives. Some is welcome; some is unwelcome; some is unplanned; some we plan and make happen. What makes our experience different from that of our ancestors, is the rate of change. It is unparalleled in history. New knowledge and technology occurs faster than our ability to apply it. Few envisioned a home computer, a VCR and a microwave oven as common household items even five years ago, nor would anyone have predicted that interest rates would change forty times or more a year. Because both our personal and work lives are affected by rapid changes, it is important to have some understanding of change itself—the kinds, the process, strategies, and how to plan and manage it.

There are basically two kinds of change, planned and unplanned. As we grow older (expected but unplanned), we begin to prepare for retirement income and housing (planned change), just as we plan to wear warmer clothing in the winter than in the summer. In addition, there is another kind of unplanned change; namely, an unanticipated result of a change such as the effect on the environment caused by the use of D.D.T.

What then, do we mean by managing change if so much is either inevitable, uncontrollable or unpredictable? There are two facets to managing change. First, when unexpected factors affect an organization, we must be prepared to alter our directions and reallocate our resources. Sometimes, one can anticipate the effects of internal or external events and prepare alternatives ahead of time. Second, if an organization is to become dynamic, it must not only incorporate **planned** change, but the expectation of planned change if it is to keep pace with new knowledge and the tools to prevent obsolescence and maintain excellence.

Indeed, planned change can also be viewed as organizational development. McGill defines organizational change as " . . . a conscious, planned process of developing an organization's capabilities so that it can attain and sustain an optimum level of performance as measured by efficiency, effectiveness and health . . . " He also notes that some organizations use a behavioral science consultant when radical changes are planned. While the reader may find that an extravagant idea, it indicates McGill's keen awareness of the necessary skills for managing change.

REACTIONS TO CHANGE

A change may represent a challenge or a threat; an opportunity for growth and improved patient satisfaction, or a disruption of accustomed tasks and relationships; a fear of failure or a chance to learn something new. Behaviors such as cooperation, compliance, open hostility or some type of subversion of the change will reflect an individual's perception of a change.

When instituting change, a manager must understand how people change and how differently each of us changes. Each person is a unique mix of genes and experiences which affect the way he or she behaves, thinks, and feels, as well as lifetime patterns of reaction, adaptation and adjustment to change.

In spite of each person's individuality, there are certain common reasons for resisting change. They are (1) a real **or** perceived threat to one's job or job relationships, (2) an unclear idea of what will be expected, (3) lack of confidence in ability to cope and succeed in the new situation and (4) loss of sense of worth. Even a desired change, such as accepting a new job promotion, can raise these specters and make us want to cling to our status quo and the known.

In an organization, such fears of the unknown will lurk to some degree in everyone, including the administrator. Stress reactions may include anger, disorganization, reduced productivity, outright refusal and illness. Other persons will turn their energies to planning, preparing themselves, finding satisfactions outside of work, physical exercise and maintain their sense of personal worth in spite of defeats.

The administrator's response to staff reactions can alter the degree of resistance, negatively or positively. It can generate more resistance if there is no self-understanding or a lack of comprehension of what employees are feeling and thinking. On the other hand, if the administrator understands the dynamics involved in change, he or she can proceed with planning not just what will be changed, but how the process of change itself will take place.

Individual responses to change may also affect organizational responses. Moore and Gergen point out the difference between organizational responses based on the kinds of employees as well as their experience with change. " . . . organizations with a history of little change probably maintain a work force of low to moderate risk takers. High risk takers would not find such an environment stimulating." They go on to say that such organizations have greater difficulty with change because greater effort must go into creating a supportive environment for the staff.

CHANGE STRATEGIES

The administrator must first assess the degree of potential impact on each part of the organization, recognizing that the change process can become emotionally charged. Then, he or she can prepare strategies for assisting individuals and groups to accommodate according to the degree of impact. While managing the change, Robert Taylor recommends that administrators begin with conceptual strategies to formulate a management approach to specific situations. A review of such strategies will make his statement more applicable.

The Empirical-Rational Strategies (described by Chin and Benne in **The Planning of Change**). These assume that people are guided by reason and self-interest. This approach suggests that giving useful information and knowledge will provide the wisdom to stimulate doing the right things. One problem with this approach is its failure to consider non-rational aspects of behavior. It is exemplified in the nursing home when we find little behavior change resulting from an inservice program. The narrowness of this approach has also been criticized in recent years because it does not adequately take into account the effect of one thing on other things (the systems approach). For instance, damming rivers on the North Pacific coast for hydroelectric power caused a deterioration of the salmon fishing industry in the Pacific Ocean. Similarly, when there was a shortage of water in San Francisco, residents were asked to conserve water; but when they used less water, the unit price to consumers went up. Thus, a rational change will first require an exploration of its possible effects on other parts of the system even though they do not appear to be affected at the time of initial consideration.

Normative Reeducation Strategies (also described by Chin and Benne). These build upon assumptions about human motivation. They relate to the attitudes, values, and beliefs that support patterns of action and practice. While rationality and intelligence are not denied in this approach, it emphasizes that changes in practice or behavior occur when persons change their value orientations and become committed to new ones. This requires that persons participate in the change process, that unconscious resistance be brought out in the open for examination and that the concepts of the behavioral sciences be used to deal with change effectively.

Power-coercive Strategies. These are a third approach to change. They are based on the use of power to effect change which may stem from the law or an influential group. Power and authority are used to gain compliance in these strategies. This is familiar to long-term care administrators. Regulatory agencies and Medicaid reimbursement systems are a part of the administrator's daily life. Medicaid legislation in the 60s changed nursing homes in radical ways for decades to come. This approach, however, can be identified in other more subtle and not so subtle situations. Power can emanate from a position, a group, a personality or by virtue of knowledge and may or may not be used appropriately. This approach may be needed when a change is selected, sanctioned, opposed or modified.

It does not, however, speak to the dynamics of implementing and managing a change within an organization unless it is used as a back-up when combined with a behavioral approach.

Havelock and Havelock describe the **social-interactive approach** to change. This approach takes into account that people influence change according to their degree of social affiliations, their influence on views held by opinion leaders and informal personal contacts. This approach might describe the political process. An administrator uses this approach when preparing a certificate of need proposal, raising funds or speaking before community groups. It begins with opinion leaders who work through networks of influence.

PLANNING THE CHANGE PROCESS

Kurt Lewin's view of the change process provides some rather specific guidelines for the administrator. His views account for the need to plan and develop change. It avoids the unwise use of power, takes time into consideration, and seems to integrate the normative re-education and social-interactive approaches. He described three phases of the change process.

Lewin's first phase, **unfreezing**, aims to prepare and motivate an individual or group for change. During this phase, the effort is to induce dissatisfaction with established practice, apply pressure to change and to restrain resisting forces while avoiding polarization. Activities during this period might include (1) circulation of pertinent readings, (2) inservice education, (3) ex-service education for a few key persons responsible for the change, (4) demonstration of change in one area or with a few residents, (5) reward of voluntary new behaviors, (6) lack of reward for old behaviors and (7) participation of staff in determining ways of achieving the goals.

Lewin's second phase is **changing or moving** from motivation to new behaviors. It occurs when there is further examination, and trying a new behavior or procedure by all parts of the system involved. First, identification of reasons for change can be focused by (1) providing a model to emulate (for example, the effect on residents), (2) setting high expectations, (3) helping people to feel safe by showing them they can succeed, and (4) increasing the attractiveness of the change. Gradually, new behaviors will become internalized and the only acceptable ones. They must be reinforced continuously by incorporating the concepts in care plans, performance appraisal systems, and informal support.

Lewin's final phase, **refreezing,** occurs when the new behavior becomes constant. It involves integration into the system, prevention of backsliding and follow-up. During this time, reinforcement should move from continuous to intermittent, policies should reflect the change, and it should be included in the orientation of personnel, families and residents. This phase culminates in a new sense of self-worth and achievement.

Dorothy Coons states that "staff will change when they have a sense of self worth." When the Geriatric wards of Michigan's Ypsilanti State Hospital were changed from a custodial to a therapeutic focus, staff had to (1) realize that their usual and established practices were obsolete, (2) learn new skills that would not reinforce long-term illness, and (3) develop new attitudes and expectations that would allow patients to improve. Coons' problems parallel those in many nursing homes. Her experience and success have applicability for nursing home administrators.

Five Principles of Helping Staff—Coons

1. Direct service staff should be involved in developing plans for change. Note, they did not decide if there would be a change, but they decided some of the "hows." Such participation prevents problems that could not be anticipated by persons removed from the immediate work situation. The staff immediately affected are best able to anticipate problems and suggest solutions.

2. "Staff must have time." They need to have time to read about new ideas, understand them, consider their effects, and get used to them. This assimilation time can be likened to that needed for a person in psychotherapy or dealing with a death. It is necessary for successful adaptation.

3. Everyone involved in an implementation plan must have a clear understanding of what it is and the steps needed to carry it out. Decisions of meetings can be put in writing and distributed in order to clarify any misunderstandings.

4. Staff should focus on developing one phase of the change at a time. This reduces disorganization from possible "overload" as described in Toffler's **Future Shock.**

5. "Staff must have opportunity to report on successes or problems." This sharing with one another can increase successes and help to

resolve any new problems more quickly than if this step does not occur.

THE ADMINISTRATOR'S ROLE

Personal Qualities

Creative long-term care requires an administrator who will assume the role of change agent as a primary responsibility. Not everyone is suited to this role because it requires an open personality, knowledge and skill in human relations, the willingness to take calculated risks, flexibility, and a sense of personal worth and confidence that is not dissipated with a failure.

The administrator who takes the change agent role seriously will select future-thinking personnel, will listen to and be influenced by those in the organization, have a natural inclination to reach out for new ideas, and realize that innovation is not the prerogative of only one person. Openness to new ideas and the ability to imagine the future also comes from exposure to a broader life: travel, history, philosophy and social activities.

Because change may produce conflict, the administrator must be knowledgeable about conflict resolution and possess negotiating skills. Thus, the administrator will be flexible in equalizing power relationships and in assigning authority and responsibility in order to produce win-win rather than win-lose results. This capacity requires well-founded trust in the character of the administrator which will be demonstrated by avoidance of coercive or devious manipulation of people.

The change agent will be committed to the need for change, comfortable with obtaining satisfaction from the successes of others, and provide staff support throughout the change process. Each planned change will lay the ground work for the next, and eventually more and more staff will begin to view change as an opportunity for personal growth and greater contribution to resident care.

Administrator Tasks in the Change Process

When an organizational change has been decided upon, the administrator needs to reflect upon the change process before implementation begins. This is necessary regardless of who initiated the idea for change and for many seemingly small as well as large changes. The following guidelines are suggested:

1. Planning
   a. Clearly state objectives in writing so that others understand where they are going.
   b. Assign resources (time, dollars, materials, personnel, etc.).
2. Assessing
   a. Who will be affected (departments, personnel, residents, families, others)?
   b. What variety of responses might be anticipated and why?
   c. Who will be supportive? Who will be unsupportive?
   d. What can be done to assist those involved during the change process?
3. Communicating
   a. Share objectives and discuss plans.
   b. Encourage suggestions and modifications by those involved.
   c. Involve inservice personnel if new knowledge, skills or roles are required.
4. Monitoring
   a. Assess any new or continued problems.
   b. Work with others to deal with daily changes.
   c. Prepare alternative strategies for timing and methods of implementation.

The more rigid the organization, of course, the greater the likelihood of resistance to new ideas. Creative organizations are more flexible and embrace a greater range of internal diversity. Indeed, diversity is a critical resource of creative organizations, but the administrator must learn how to use it so that it does not result in polarization of individuals and groups. Creative organizations have special characteristics (Schaller). They include the following:

1. The administrator recognizes that conflict is a part of the creative change process, but that polarization can be a barrier to planned change. Thus the administrator:
   a. Keeps communication channels open.
   b. Attempts to depersonalize dissent.
   c. Attempts to identify the needs and fears of others.
   d. Encourages meaningful participation in planning by every person involved.

    e. Begins by seeking agreement on short-term or intermediate goals.

    f. Builds a sense of trust throughout the organization.

2. The primary organizational focus is on contemporary practice, not that of yesterday or perpetuation of the organization.

3. There is constant awareness that problems do exist.

4. The emphasis is on problem solving.

5. There is emphasis on locating important and relevant knowledge from a variety of disciplines and "an unusual flare for utilizing and applying the knowledge, wisdom, and insights of other disciplines."

6. Continuous monitoring of the benefits and pace of change prevent the possibility of too much disruption.

7. When new ideas are proposed, the leader knows the most receptive points of intervention.

In summary, the administrator needs to continually monitor the pulse of the change process. Is it too fast? Can it be speeded up? Do certain individuals require special attention (counseling, reassurance, education, etc.)? What can be done to maintain participation, maintain movement toward the new goals and support those involved during the process?

If long-term care organizations are to develop their capabilities, and at the same time maintain their missions and services, organizational viability and productivity, the administrator must become a change agent. Changes can be successful and foster growth in organizational outcomes if the administrator understands not just the goals and mechanics of a change but management of the change process itself.

REFERENCES AND RESOURCES

Bennis, W. G., K. D. Benne, R. Chin, and K. E. Correy. *The Planning of Change*, 3rd ed., New York, Holt, Rinehart and Winston, 1976.

Coons, Dorothy. *The Process of Change*, Ann Arbor, Institute of Gerontology, University of Michigan, 1973.

Gergen, Paul and Maggie Moore. "Risk Taking and Organizational Change," *Training and Development Journal*, 39:3:284, June, 1985.

Hallett, J. "Today's Trends Suggest Revolutionary Changes for Business in the Future," *Personnel Administrator*, 30:2:64–74, 1985.

Havelock, R. G. and M. C. Havelock. *Training for Change Agents*, Institute of Social Research, Ann Arbor, MI 1973.

Kanter, Rosabeth Moss. *The Change Masters: Innovating for Productivity in the American Corporation*, New York, Simon & Schuster, 1983.

McGill, Michael E. *Organizational Development for Operating Managers,* New York, AMACOM, 1977.

Peters, Joseph P. and Simone Tseng. "Managing Strategic Change: Moving Others from Awareness to Action," *Hospital & Health Services Administration,* July/August, 1984, p. 60.

Schaller, Lyle E., *The Change Agent,* Nashville, Abington Press, 1972.

Taylor, Robert and Tom Dogloff. *The Management of Change,* a monograph, Minneapolis, University of Minnesota, Division of Health Services Administration, 1987.

Tichy, Noel. *Managing Strategic Change: Technical, Political and Cultural Dynamics,* New York, John Wiley, 1983.

Toffler, Alvin. *Future Shock,* New York, Random House, 1970.

APPENDIX A

GUIDELINES FOR A
NONDISCRIMINATORY APPLICATION FORM

There is a variety of state and federal laws which are aimed at preventing discriminatory practices by employers. Generally speaking, they relate to age, sex, race or color, religion, national origin, and physical disability. It is strongly recommended that you check the wording and all information requested on your application form with your State Employment Office. Your lawyer, of course, can be consulted also. The following suggestions have been prepared to assist in formulating a nondiscriminatory application form.

Item	Recommendation
Religion	Omit
Race or Color	Omit
Sex	Omit
Sexual preference	Omit
Marital status	Omit
Number of children	Omit—You may wish to ask, "Do you have any responsibilities that will interfere with your ability to be prompt and reliable in attendance?"
Birthplace	Omit—Ask, "Are you a U.S. citizen?" If no, "Does your visa prohibit you from working here?"
Age	Omit—Ask, "Are you between 18 and 70 years of age? If not, what is your age?"
Disabilities	"Do you have any physical, mental or medical disability which would interfere with performing the job for which you are applying?"
Next of kin	Omit—emergency numbers can be obtained if the applicant is employed.
Height and weight	Omit
Arrest record	Omit—You may ask, "Have you ever been convicted of a crime? If so, give details."
Education	Ask, "highest grade attained and dates of any vocational, professional or academic education."
Finances or bills owed	Omit

321

Military experience	Omit any question about type of discharge. Ask, "Have you served in any U.S. military service? Describe the training and experience gained there."
Photograph	Omit, but state that a photograph may be required after employment if this is the case.
References	"Names of persons willing to provide character or work references. Please initial names you are willing to have us contact."

NAME INDEX

SUBJECT INDEX